MINDFULNESS-BASED THERAPY
FOR INSOMNIA

MINDFULNESS-BASED THERAPY
FOR INSOMNIA

JASON C. ONG

American Psychological Association • Washington, DC

Published by
American Psychological Association
750 First Street, NE
Washington, DC 20002
www.apa.org

To order
APA Order Department
P.O. Box 92984
Washington, DC 20090-2984
Tel: (800) 374-2721; Direct: (202) 336-5510
Fax: (202) 336-5502; TDD/TTY: (202) 336-6123
Online: www.apa.org/pubs/books
E-mail: order@apa.org

In the U.K., Europe, Africa, and the Middle East, copies may be ordered from
American Psychological Association
3 Henrietta Street
Covent Garden, London
WC2E 8LU England

Typeset in Meridien by Circle Graphics, Inc., Columbia, MD

Printer: United Book Press, Baltimore, MD
Cover Designer: Mercury Publishing Services, Inc., Rockville, MD

The opinions and statements published are the responsibility of the authors, and such opinions and
statements do not necessarily represent the policies of the American Psychological Association.

Library of Congress Cataloging-in-Publication Data

Names: Ong, Jason C., author.
Title: Mindfulness-based therapy for insomnia / Jason C. Ong.
Description: Washington, DC : American Psychological Association, [2017] |
  Includes bibliographical references and index.
Identifiers: LCCN 2016009048 | ISBN 9781433822414 | ISBN 1433822415
Subjects: LCSH: Insomnia—Treatment. | Mindfulness-based cognitive therapy.
Classification: LCC RC548 .O54 2017 | DDC 616.8/49820651—dc23
LC record available at http://lccn.loc.gov/2016009048

British Library Cataloguing-in-Publication Data
A CIP record is available from the British Library.

Printed in the United States of America
First Edition

http://dx.doi.org/10.1037/14952-000

This book is dedicated to three psychologists who recently passed away:
Richard Bootzin, Arthur Spielman, and Peter Hauri.
Their work in insomnia inspired me to pursue specialized training in sleep,
and I hope to build on the foundation they created.

Contents

Preface

have spent most of my professional career as a scientist–practitioner, trying to carve out a research niche in behavioral clinical trials while hoping to help people sleep better. I never imagined that I would have the opportunity to write a book that could bring the concepts of mindfulness meditation to work with the problems of chronic insomnia.

When this opportunity first presented itself, it was overwhelming trying to fit the research findings and the lessons learned into one neat product. This struggle led to reflections on why this work is important and how things came together for this project. Looking back, my journey to discovering mindfulness and sleep was built on some personal struggles and many fortunate opportunities.

On a personal level, I have experienced chronic insomnia and the frustration of not being able to control sleep. This began when I was in grade school, well before I had any formal training in psychology, mindfulness meditation, or behavioral sleep medicine. Perhaps it was the struggle with sleep at an early age that reinforced my interest in mind–body relationships and finding different approaches to problems that appeared uncontrollable. In my eighth-grade biology class, I even wrote an essay on insomnia. Perhaps prophetic, the essay was on nonpharmacological treatments for insomnia.

My clinical training was oriented in cognitive-behavioral approaches and I learned to deliver cognitive behavior therapy for insomnia (CBT-I) during my clinical internship and postdoctoral fellowship. I really enjoyed this work and found it very rewarding to help people sleep better without using drugs. However, some patients did not respond to CBT-I and felt even more hopeless when they did not have immediate success. To some of them, the behavioral strategies seemed to involve a method of forced sleep deprivation and "toughing out" the daytime consequences by not taking naps. At times, I found it difficult to convince unwilling patients to change their sleep schedule and bedtime routine or to engage in cognitive restructuring about their sleep. Although I believed in the components of CBT-I, it was difficult as a young therapist to work with the resistance from these challenging patients. I wondered whether there was another way to deliver some of these components in a more experiential and compassionate context.

Dr. Rachel Manber was my primary mentor during my postdoctoral fellowship at Stanford University. Dr. Manber was also trained as a cognitive behavior therapist, but she often took a more compassionate approach to delivering CBT-I. She could detect a patient's frustration and disappointment when sleep did not improve, and she would suggest a more accepting, nonjudging approach, rather than trying to push the behavioral strategies. Dr. Manber introduced the concepts of mindfulness to me and showed how it could be applied to working with insomnia patients. She also encouraged me to connect with other experts in mindfulness meditation to stimulate my thinking about using that method as an approach to insomnia. As I received further training in mindfulness meditation, I realized how much it connected with my personal interest in Eastern philosophy. I had a minor in philosophy as an undergraduate, and I had read many books on Zen Buddhism as well as the teachings of the Dalai Lama. Dr. Manber provided the genesis of the idea for using mindfulness to improve our current treatments for insomnia, as she had been informally using mindfulness techniques at the Stanford Sleep Clinic but had not yet conducted formal research to test the use of mindfulness for insomnia. Under Dr. Manber's mentorship, we decided to embark on a journey to develop and test a treatment program using mindfulness meditation for insomnia, which we now call *mindfulness-based therapy for insomnia* (MBTI).

We started testing MBTI in California, which seemed like a place where people would be open to meditation and integrative medicine. When I later moved to Chicago, I was uncertain how the idea would be received. I was pleasantly surprised to find that the interest was strong, which paralleled an overall rising interest in using mindfulness-based approaches to improve health. After publishing our research studies on MBTI, I began receiving requests from patients, clinicians, and media outlets who wanted to learn more about MBTI.

This book describes the principles and practices of MBTI and the research that has been conducted on MBTI. Writing this book itself has been a practice in mindfulness. Many times during the writing process, I felt our work was incomplete, and I had to practice nonjudging and letting go of my own attachment to writing the perfect book. Alas, this book is not a perfect product but a work in progress—and I hope readers will continue the progress that we began.

Acknowledgments

There are many people to thank who directly and indirectly contributed to this book. First, I would like to thank the mentors and advisors who have guided me on this journey. Rachel Manber is one of the most talented people I have ever met, and this book would never have been written without her contributions and mentorship. I would also like to thank several other mentors: Shauna Shapiro, a professor at Santa Clara University, whose mentorship on mindfulness and health has been invaluable in helping to shape the concepts in mindfulness-based therapy for insomnia (MBTI) as well as my personal mindfulness practices; James Wyatt for his mentorship on sleep and circadian physiology as well as guidance on managing clinical trials; Bob Stahl, who trains mindfulness-based stress reduction (MBSR) teachers in California and helped shape how I lead meditations and encouraged me to grow deeper in my understanding of mindfulness concepts and my own personal practice; and Zindel Segal, who provided mentorship on research and clinical issues related to developing MBTI on the basis of the wisdom he gained from developing mindfulness-based cognitive therapy. I would also like to thank Edward Stepanski, Sandy Gramling, and Roseanne Armitage for their mentorship early in my training.

I would also like to thank those who have contributed to our research projects: David Sholtes and Christina Khou, our project coordinators; Isabel Crisostomo, our medical director; and those who served as instructors and therapists in our research studies: Arthur Hoffman, Vered Hankin, Jamie Cvengros, Megan Hood, Jamie Jackson, Heather Gunn, Liisa Hantsoo, Mark Neenan, and Sharon Allen. Special thanks to Megan Crawford and Eric Schmidt, who reviewed early drafts of this book and provided helpful comments. I also want to thank Susan Reynolds, David Becker, Liz Brace, Ron Teeter, and the team at APA Books for their guidance and support throughout the writing of this book. Your help was invaluable for a first-time author.

I want to acknowledge the research grant support that I received from the National Center for Complementary and Integrative Health to carry out the research studies on MBTI and MBSR.

Finally, I want to thank my family for supporting me during this journey; especially my wife, Amye, whose love and partnership inspires me to make value-congruent decisions in our journey together.

MINDFULNESS-BASED THERAPY
FOR INSOMNIA

Introduction

Sleep is an essential part of life that most people take for granted. We assume that the mind and the body will naturally "turn off" when we decide to lie down in bed and rest. After about 8 hours of sleep, we feel refreshed, we get out of bed, and we "turn on" the mind and the body to start our day. This routine sounds simple, like putting a computer in low-energy mode when not in use and then booting it up when needed. However, sleep does not always occur when we decide it should happen. Sometimes the mind will not shut off, or the body is restless and unable to power down. Wakefulness invades the bed, like an intruder in the night. If the inability to sleep persists, it can lead to tension, anxiety, and desperate attempts to shut off the mind and body. Unfortunately, these efforts are usually ineffective. This pattern is well-known to people with chronic insomnia.

Sleeplessness is a highly prevalent health problem, with about one third to one half of adults reporting regular difficulty falling asleep or staying asleep, and about 7% to 18% of

http://dx.doi.org/10.1037/14952-001

Mindfulness-Based Therapy for Insomnia, by J. C. Ong

adults meeting criteria for an insomnia disorder (Jansson-Fröjmark & Linton, 2008; Ohayon, 2002; LeBlanc et al., 2009). Sleep disturbance can impair cognitive functioning, compromise immune functioning, and exacerbate psychiatric conditions. The economic impact of insomnia-related absenteeism has been estimated to have an annual indirect cost of $970.6 million, and insomnia-related productivity losses are estimated at $5 billion (Daley, Morin, LeBlanc, Grégoire, & Savard, 2009).

When acute sleep disturbance goes untreated, it can evolve into a chronic insomnia disorder, which consists of sleep-specific symptoms (e.g., difficulty falling and staying asleep) associated with significant waking distress or impairment. Although the initial sleep disturbance is often triggered or precipitated by a stress response, development of chronic insomnia involves responses to the sleep disturbance that inadvertently dysregulate sleep physiology and perpetuate a state of mental and physical hyperarousal. These responses include behavioral changes, such as staying in bed to sleep in or taking naps, or using substances, such as sleep medication or caffeine. Furthermore, increased effort to sleep might also increase cognitive-emotional distress related to sleep by developing maladaptive beliefs and attitudes about sleep, rigid expectations about sleep, and increased attention given to figuring out how to sleep. All of these can create a vicious cycle of insomnia that is encapsulated by hyperarousal.

Pharmacological treatments can be effective short-term treatments, but side effects, such as amnestic episodes, are reported by patients. Furthermore, many patients still experience sleep disturbance despite taking these drugs, leading to dependence on and tolerance of the drugs. The leading nonpharmacological treatment is cognitive behavior therapy for insomnia (CBT-I), which has substantial evidence to support treatment effectiveness. However, the current cadre of qualified providers cannot meet the demand of the number of people who suffer from insomnia, and there are still many people who do not respond to CBT-I. Developing other empirically supported treatment options can provide more choices for consumers.

What Is Mindfulness-Based Therapy for Insomnia, and Why Is It Needed?

This book describes the principles and practices of a new treatment program for insomnia called *mindfulness-based therapy for insomnia* (MBTI). This integrative treatment package brings together the principles and practices of mindfulness meditation with some of the behavioral strategies used in CBT-I. Mindfulness meditation is a form of Buddhist meditation that focuses on present-moment awareness as a means to see with discernment, cultivate self-compassion, and relieve one's suffering. The practice of mindfulness involves awareness of the impermanence of nature, including the observation that thoughts in the mind are not facts of reality but mental events that are dynamic rather than static. By choosing to become aware of whatever is present in the mind and reconceptualizing thoughts and desires as mental events that simply come and go, one can let go of the attachment to these thoughts and desires. This mental process is called *metacognitive shifting* and is one of the keys to reducing the stress and effort put into trying to sleep better in the MBTI program.

MBTI was originally developed by Rachel Manber, Shauna Shapiro, and me, refined with input from Zindel Segal. We developed MBTI not because we thought a new, better insomnia treatment was needed but because we recognized that most people who suffer from insomnia try too hard to solve their "sleep problem." We wanted to help sufferers of insomnia see the problem in a different way and to provide some tools to help them sleep better at night and function better during the day. We felt that teaching mindfulness meditation could provide an opportunity to create the space needed to allow sleep to come back. Through meditation practice, patients with insomnia can learn from their own thoughts, feelings, and sensations with an MBTI teacher as their guide.

The MBTI program is designed as an eight-session group intervention with an optional meditation retreat in between the later sessions. Each session is approximately 2.5 hours and consists of the following three activities: (a) formal meditations, (b) period of discussion, and (c) insomnia-related activities and instructions. Each week consists of a theme involving principles of mindfulness integrated with behavioral sleep medicine along with the practices of mindfulness meditation and behavioral strategies for sleep. In addition to activities in session, participants are assigned home meditation practice, starting from the first session. The type of meditation practice assigned varies according to the lessons and meditations that are taught during the session that week. Typically, participants are assigned to practice meditations for at least 30 minutes, 6 days per week. To aid in the home meditation practice, guided meditations using digital media are provided along with a log or diary to record their meditation practice and sleep patterns.

Research studies have provided empirical support for the efficacy of MBTI. A randomized controlled trial revealed that MBTI was superior to a self-monitoring control in decreasing self-reported total wake time in bed, decreasing presleep arousal, and reducing symptoms of insomnia (Ong et al., 2014). Furthermore, patients can achieve clinically meaningful benefits from MBTI with a rate of response of 60% at posttreatment and 79% at 6-month follow-up. Similar results were found for remission, with a 33% remission rate at posttreatment and a 50% remission rate at 6-month follow-up for MBTI. When compared with mindfulness-based stress reduction, the standard mindfulness-based therapy, MBTI was superior in decreasing insomnia symptoms from baseline to 6-month follow-up.

A Road Map for Using This Book

This book is designed primarily for clinicians and trainees in psychology, psychiatry, medicine, nursing, and social work who work with individuals suffering from chronic insomnia or who wish to expand their practice into this area. It is also intended for teachers of mindfulness-based therapies who have appropriate credentials for working with clinical populations and are interested in expanding their work to people who have insomnia. Researchers and scholars will also find this book to be a useful resource for summarizing the research literature on MBTI and other mindfulness-based approaches for insomnia. Given the wide audience and range of potential practitioners, I have used the term *instructor* rather than *therapist* or *teacher* when referring to the individual delivering MBTI.

This book is organized into three parts. Part I provides the reader with a background on insomnia and the principles of mindfulness meditation to provide a context for understanding MBTI and its contents. Chapter 1 presents an overview of insomnia, with definitions and terms that are used throughout the book and in discussions of the scope of the problem. Chapter 2 describes the current pharmacological and nonpharmacological treatment options, with a discussion of the benefits and limitations of these treatments. Chapter 3 describes the principles and origins of mindfulness meditation to serve as a background for understanding the application of mindfulness to the problem of insomnia.

Part II features the theory and content of the MBTI program. The title, Principles and Practices of MBTI, was selected to emphasize the practice of meditation as a core feature of MBTI. Structurally, this section provides direct guidance to clinicians who are interested in delivering MBTI, including session-by-session program materials and instructions for delivering specific treatment components. Some readers might find it helpful to refer back to Part I as they encounter parts of MBTI that refer to sleep physiology or mindfulness principles. Chapter 4 presents the application of mindfulness principles to insomnia and the metacognitive model of insomnia that serve as the theoretical basis for MBTI. The next four chapters provide detailed descriptions of the contents for each MBTI session, including session outlines and guidance for leading meditations and other in-session activities. Sample handouts that accompany these sessions can be found in the Appendix. Chapter 5 discusses the activities in Sessions 1 and 2, focusing on how to get started with MBTI. Chapter 6 describes Sessions 3 and 4, focusing on establishing the meditation practice and delivering the behavioral strategies for insomnia. Chapter 7 highlights the tools and activities for making metacognitive changes that are used in Sessions 5, 6, and 7. Chapter 8 describes the activities for bringing MBTI to closure in Session 8 and provides some suggestions for handling challenges that can occur while delivering MBTI. After reading this section, clinicians should understand the principles of MBTI, the skills needed to effectively deliver MBTI, and the materials that are needed throughout the MBTI program.

Part III discusses the empirical evidence for using mindfulness as a treatment for insomnia and considerations for implementing MBTI in real-world practice. Chapter 9 presents the program of research involved in developing and testing MBTI and the research base on other mindfulness-based therapies for insomnia. Researchers might be particularly interested in this chapter, which presents considerations and strategic decisions we made regarding research methodology. Chapter 10 broadens the discussion to consider how MBTI fits into the real world of health care delivery, with discussions on issues related to patient considerations and provider competency. Resources for further reading and training on mindfulness and insomnia are included in Chapter 10 to help guide instructors who are interested in delivering MBTI.

Insomnia is a widespread but treatable condition, and further efforts are needed to address this public health issue. The American Psychological Association (APA) recently recognized sleep psychology as a specialty, acknowledging the important role that psychologists can play in treating sleep disorders. My hope for this book is that it will bring the principles and practices of MBTI to a wider audience of clinicians, which can expand treatment options for people suffering from insomnia. Although I have previously published the research findings in scientific journals and presented workshops on MBTI at scientific meetings, this book provides details about the delivery of MBTI and describes the decisions that were made in putting the treatment package together. The materials include handouts and instructions that should enable clinicians with proper training to begin delivering MBTI. Other resources such as videos, workshops, and professional continuing education courses can be used to supplement this book. In addition, I hope that the contents of this book will stimulate clinical researchers to consider new ways to improve MBTI, to study the treatment mechanisms, and to investigate other populations that could benefit from this treatment approach. Overall, I hope that the information in this book can provide the reader with novel ways to conceptualize insomnia and help those suffering from this common sleep disorder.

BACKGROUND

Insomnia
The Problem of Sleeplessness

1

This chapter provides an overview of *insomnia*, a sleep disorder characterized by sleeplessness and unwanted wakefulness in bed. First, the current diagnostic criteria are reviewed, along with the definitions and terms used in this book. Next, the epidemiology and etiology of insomnia are presented to indicate the scope of this disorder and the significance of its impact on the individual and society. The concepts on sleep and insomnia from this chapter serve as important background information that mindfulness-based therapy for insomnia (MBTI) instructors should master prior to delivering MBTI.

http://dx.doi.org/10.1037/14952-002
Mindfulness-Based Therapy for Insomnia, by J. C. Ong

What Is Insomnia?

CHARACTERIZING INSOMNIA: DEFINITIONS AND TERMS

Is insomnia a distinct disorder, or is it just a symptom of a more serious condition? This fundamental question has been debated by clinicians, researchers, and those experiencing sleep problems. In most lay contexts, *insomnia* is a term that generally refers to "not sleeping well." This might include difficulty falling asleep at the beginning of the night, waking up in the middle of the night and having difficulty falling back to sleep, or waking too early and having difficulty sleeping until the desired wake-up time. These are symptoms of sleep disturbance that cause an individual to have insufficient sleep. However, these symptoms are also experienced in the course of everyday living, such as during a stressful period. Many people who experience these symptoms on occasion do not seek treatment until the symptoms begin to affect daytime functioning. Moreover, these symptoms alone do not provide specificity in terms of the need for treatment or the consequences arising from prolonged sleep disturbance. Thus, in the clinical context, insomnia rises to a distinct and diagnosable disorder when the sleep-specific symptoms are associated with symptoms that occur while awake, including distress about not sleeping or functional impairment related to insufficient sleep. Examples of waking distress or impairment include excessive sleepiness or fatigue, difficulty maintaining attention or concentration, and mood disturbances. Therefore, the term *insomnia* could refer to either symptoms of sleep disturbance (i.e., difficulty falling asleep, staying asleep, or early morning awakenings) or a distinct disorder. This conceptualization of the term *insomnia* as consisting of either symptoms or a disorder was recommended by a workgroup led by Buysse, Ancoli-Israel, Edinger, Lichstein, and Morin (2006) as part of the recommendations for standardization of insomnia assessment. In this book, the term *insomnia* is used to refer to an insomnia disorder (unless otherwise indicated).

A second question to consider is the timing of the sleep disturbance. Does it matter if the complaint is with sleep onset (i.e., difficulty falling asleep), sleep maintenance (i.e., difficulty falling back to sleep in the middle of the night), or early morning awakenings? The accumulated literature has not found that patients with these distinctions of sleep disturbances respond differently to treatments for insomnia. Therefore, the differences in the location of the sleep disturbance are typically referred to as *insomnia phenotypes*, denoting different presentations in the timing of sleep disturbance that stem from a common insomnia disorder. This characterization of insomnia phenotypes is also used in this book.

Another controversial area involves quantitative cutoffs for defining the threshold for insomnia. How long does it have to take one to
fall asleep before it is considered abnormal and a sign of insomnia?
Also, how frequently does the sleep disturbance need to occur? It is
interesting to note that people with insomnia frequently operate on
the assumption that normal sleepers fall asleep immediately. However,
falling asleep too quickly can be an indication of insufficient sleep or
another type of sleep disorder, such as narcolepsy. Lichstein, Durrence,
Taylor, Bush, and Riedel (2003) examined the sensitivity and specificity
of different criteria based on sleep diary data. The authors found that a
cutoff score for either sleep onset latency (SOL) or wake time after sleep
onset (WASO) of 31 minutes or more occurring three or more times
per week was the optimal quantitative criteria for insomnia. Another
study found that a cutoff score of 20 minutes or more over a 2-week
period was the optimal criteria for maximizing sensitivity and specificity (Lineberger, Carney, Edinger, & Means, 2006). Given the subjective
nature of sleep diary data, quantitative data have not been uniformly
adopted in research or diagnostic classification systems. However, many
clinicians and researchers will use SOL or WASO longer than 30 minutes
as an indicator of a clinically significant amount of wakefulness in bed.

CLASSIFICATION OF INSOMNIA DISORDERS

The current diagnostic systems have generally adopted these terms and
concepts for insomnia. In the fifth edition of the *Diagnostic and Statistical
Manual for Mental Disorders* (*DSM–5*; American Psychiatric Association,
2013), the diagnostic criteria for an insomnia disorder include a predominant complaint of dissatisfaction with sleep quantity or quality
(difficulty initiating sleep, difficulty maintaining sleep, or early morning
awakenings) that causes clinically significant distress or impairment. The
sleep difficulty must occur three or more times per week for 3 or more
months and be present despite adequate opportunity for sleep. Further
specification of the insomnia disorder is included if the insomnia disorder is comorbid with another mental, medical, or sleep disorder. Specification is also included for episodic (symptoms occur for 1 month or more
but for less than 3 months), persistent (for 3 months or more), or recurrent insomnia (two or more episodes within 1 year). The *International
Classification System of Sleep Disorders—Third Edition* (*ICSD–3*; American
Academy of Sleep Medicine, 2014) has very similar diagnostic criteria
but distinguishes chronic insomnia disorder as an insomnia disorder
that is present for 3 months or more and short-term (or adjustment)
insomnia if the symptoms of the insomnia disorder have been present
for less than 3 months. In this book, we have adopted these criteria to
refer to insomnia disorders, unless otherwise specified. Furthermore,

the evidence base for MBTI is generally consistent with these criteria for insomnia (see Chapter 9, this volume, for an in-depth discussion).

These criteria reflect a shift in the conceptualization of insomnia. Early conceptualizations considered sleep disturbance (i.e., insomnia symptoms) to be only a symptom of an underlying disorder, most typically a mood or anxiety disorder. This led to underrecognition of insomnia as a treatable disorder because treatments at that time were focused on resolving the "underlying disorder." However, many people continued to experience persistent insomnia even when the underling disorder was controlled. As the field of sleep medicine emerged, the classification began to shift toward categorization of primary and secondary insomnia. In the fourth edition of the *DSM* (*DSM–IV*; American Psychiatric Association, 2000), primary and secondary insomnia were diagnosed based on the attribution of the cause of the insomnia symptoms. Primary insomnia was diagnosed when the insomnia symptoms were clinically significant and not related to another condition, thus requiring independent treatment. The second edition of the *International Classification of Sleep Disorders* (American Academy of Sleep Medicine, 2005) further distinguished subtypes of primary insomnia on the basis of presumed etiology, including psychophysiological insomnia, paradoxical insomnia, idiopathic insomnia, and inadequate sleep hygiene. Secondary insomnia was diagnosed when the insomnia symptoms were related to another medical or psychiatric condition. As a result, the insomnia symptoms were presumed to resolve with successful treatment of the underlying condition. Although this distinction clarified clinical decision making related to the treatment of insomnia, it was soon realized that clinicians were not very accurate at discerning when insomnia was independent from another condition. A study examining patterns of diagnosis across different clinics using the *DSM–IV* and *ICSD* found that insomnia related to another mental disorder was the most common diagnosis in 44% of cases, and primary insomnia was the second most common diagnosis in about 20% of cases (Buysse et al., 1994). More recently, a creative study by Edinger et al. (2011) using a multitrait, multimethod design found that clinicians were not very reliable at discerning the causes of insomnia related to subtypes or distinguishing primary versus secondary insomnia. These findings were very influential for the shift from a "splitting" to a "lumping" approach for classifying insomnia disorders. In the *DSM–5* and *ICSD–3*, an insomnia disorder is diagnosed without the distinction between primary and secondary insomnia.

Starting in October 2015, the Affordable Care Act mandated the use of the *International Classification of Diseases, Tenth Revision, Clinical Modification* (*ICD–10–CM*; Buck, 2015; see http://www.cdc.gov/nchs/icd/icd10cm.htm) for diagnostic and procedure coding in the United States. This coding system includes a wide range of codes for diseases and other features (e.g., signs, symptoms, circumstances, external causes of injury or diseases) that provide more detail and allow for greater specificity in tracking health care data. For the diagnosis of insomnia disorders, the *ICD–10–CM* does not contain any new criteria, but it does introduce new diagnostic codes that represent a combination of the ICSD and *DSM* classifications. For example, chronic insomnia disorder in the *ICSD–3* is now classified as primary insomnia (e.g., F51.01) in the *ICD–10–CM*. In contrast to the *ICSD–3* and *DSM–5*, the *ICD–10–CM* assigns separate codes to certain subtypes of insomnia. For example, the *ICD–10–CM* includes a code for psychophysiological insomnia (e.g., F51.04), a subtype of insomnia from the second edition of the *ICSD*, in which elevated arousal is a distinguishing feature. It is not clear why the *ICD–10–CM* did not update the codes to match the lumping approach taken in the *ICSD–3* and *DSM–5*.

Epidemiology of Insomnia

HOW COMMON IS INSOMNIA?

The challenges in defining insomnia have also created challenges in studying its epidemiology. The variations in how insomnia was defined and assessed led to a wide range of estimates of how many people were afflicted with this condition, ranging from as little as 6% of the population to over 50% of the general adult population (National Sleep Foundation, 2002; Ohayon, 2002). Ohayon (2002) provided a very useful illustration of summarizing the epidemiological literature using the distinctions between insomnia symptoms and disorder and diagnostic criteria (see Figure 1.1). As depicted in Figure 1.1, Ohayon used a funnel to illustrate how the prevalence of insomnia in adults changed with the definition of insomnia. At the top, a broad definition of insomnia using just symptoms resulted in a rather broad prevalence between 30% and 48%. As the criteria became stricter, to include daytime consequences, dissatisfaction with the sleep quality or quantity, and meeting an insomnia diagnosis (ruling out other differential diagnoses), the prevalence dropped and became more precise, funneling toward a prevalence of 6% when using *DSM–IV* criteria. These numbers are relatively consistent with other epidemiological studies that have used longitudinal data. One study, conducted on over 400 adults in Canada, found that the 1-year incidence rates of insomnia symptoms were 30.7% and 7.4% for an insomnia syndrome, which were closely related to the definitions of an insomnia disorder (LeBlanc et al., 2009). Another study, conducted on more than 1,700 adults in Sweden, measured symptoms of insomnia at two time points 1 year apart

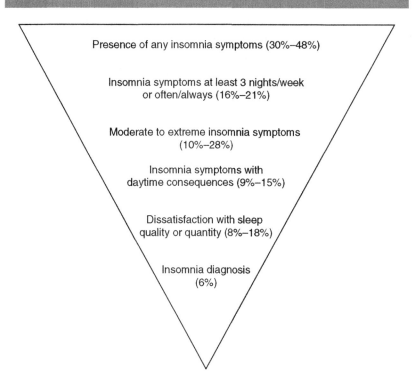

Presence of any insomnia symptoms (30%–48%)

Insomnia symptoms at least 3 nights/week
or often/always (16%–21%)

Moderate to extreme insomnia symptoms
(10%–28%)

Insomnia symptoms with
daytime consequences (9%–15%)

Dissatisfaction with sleep
quality or quantity (8%–18%)

Insomnia diagnosis
(6%)

Percentage of individuals who endorsed symptoms of sleep disturbance and daytime dysfunction related to criteria for insomnia. From "Epidemiology of Insomnia: What We Know and What We Still Need to Learn," by M. M. Ohayon, 2002, *Sleep Medicine Reviews*, 6, p. 100. Copyright 2002 by Elsevier. Adapted with permission.

(Jansson-Fröjmark & Linton, 2008). The authors found that the cross-sectional prevalence of an insomnia disorder was 6.8% at baseline and 9.7% at the 1-year follow-up, with 44% of those reporting insomnia at baseline also reporting insomnia at follow-up. This corresponded to 4.3% of the population that reported a persistent insomnia disorder. The persistence of insomnia was also documented in a longitudinal 3-year study examining the natural history of insomnia (Morin et al., 2009). Examining nearly 400 adults in the general population, Morin and colleagues (2009) found that 46% of the sample reported insomnia persisting over the 3-year period, with persistent insomnia associated with more severe insomnia at baseline, among women, and at an older age. Moreover, 27% of those who experienced remission of insomnia during the 3-year study also experienced a relapse of insomnia. In summary, at any given time, about one third to one half of adults will report symptoms of insomnia, and about 6% to 10% of the population will meet criteria for an insomnia disorder. Furthermore, a little less than one half of adults with an insomnia disorder will experience a chronic (or persistent) insomnia disorder over the course of 1 to 3 years. These epidemiological findings highlight the broad impact of insomnia across the population and the persistence of this sleep disorder across time.

RISK FACTORS FOR INSOMNIA

Several demographic and socioeconomic factors can moderate the risk of developing insomnia. Women are about 1.4 times more likely than men to report insomnia symptoms (Ohayon, 2002). The reasons for the gender differences are unclear, but hormonal factors related to menopause have been hypothesized to play a role, given that postmenopausal women report higher levels of insomnia compared with premenopausal women (Ohayon, 2002). Age is another key risk factor, with up to 50% of older adults over age 65 reporting symptoms of insomnia (Ohayon, 2002). Although there are some intrinsic changes in sleep related to the process of aging, insomnia in older adults appears to be more closely related to daytime behaviors such as inactivity or social dissatisfaction and the presence of comorbid medical and psychiatric disorders rather than the natural aging process (Ohayon, Zulley, Guilleminault, Smirne, & Priest, 2001). With regard to the phenotype of insomnia, middle-aged and older adults report more difficulty with sleep maintenance, whereas adolescents and younger adults are more likely to report difficulty falling asleep. Beyond gender and age, there is some evidence that insomnia can occur at more elevated rates among those with a family history of insomnia, individuals with lower income levels, and those who are not employed. However, the findings are not clear, especially because the key risk factors of gender and age are often not adequately controlled in these studies.

ASSOCIATED COMORBID CONDITIONS

As noted earlier, insomnia can co-occur with another condition or disorder. The most commonly associated mental disorder is unipolar depression (Breslau, Roth, Rosenthal, & Andreski, 1996; Ford & Kamerow, 1989); anxiety disorders are also highly prevalent, although the specific type of anxiety disorder is not consistently related to insomnia across studies (Breslau et al., 1996). Substance use, including alcohol and nicotine use, is also commonly associated with insomnia. In terms of medical conditions, insomnia often occurs in the context of cancer, chronic pain, heart disease, pulmonary diseases, and gastrointestinal diseases (D. J. Taylor et al., 2007). One study found a dose–response relationship between the number of medical conditions and the complaint of insomnia among older adults (ages 55–84) in the United States (Foley, Ancoli-Israel, Britz, & Walsh, 2004). The prevalence of older adults who reported at least one symptom of insomnia rose from 36% (among those who did not endorse any medical conditions) to 52% (among older adults who endorsed one to three medical conditions), to 69% (among older adults who endorsed four or more medical conditions). Finally, insomnia can be associated with another sleep disorder, such as obstructive sleep apnea or restless legs syndrome. Careful assessment of the severity of the sleep disturbance and the relationship among symptoms of insomnia and the other sleep disorder is needed to determine whether an insomnia disorder is indeed present. In general, if an insomnia disorder can be diagnosed—even when a comorbid condition is present—then treatment for insomnia should be initiated. If left untreated, insomnia can be highly related to other negative health consequences. Therefore, treatment of insomnia is important in the context of a comorbid condition.

CONSEQUENCES OF INSOMNIA

Having insomnia is more than a nuisance. There are very real functional, biological, and emotional consequences that can have deleterious effects on health, quality of life, and productivity. First, insomnia can impair cognitive functioning. Although the literature has shown mixed results, a few general patterns have emerged recently. In the context of insomnia, cognitive impairments tend to occur during complex cognitive tasks, such as working memory and attention-switching tasks in which executive control plays an important role (Fernandez-Mendoza et al., 2010; Shekleton et al., 2014). In addition, these cognitive impairments are most pronounced among people with insomnia who have objectively measured short sleep duration (Edinger, Means, Carney, & Krystal, 2008; Fernandez-Mendoza et al., 2010). Furthermore, people with insomnia demonstrate a more variable pattern in response over time (Edinger et al., 2008), suggesting that efforts to "rally" cognitive resources can overcome the effects of sleep deficit in short bursts but are difficult to sustain over time.

The presence of insomnia is also associated with adverse biological consequences. Sleep disturbance can compromise immune functioning (Irwin, 2015), and insomnia is associated with cardiovascular conditions, including high blood pressure (D. J. Taylor et al., 2007; Vgontzas, Liao, Bixler, Chrousos, & Vela-Bueno, 2009). People with insomnia can develop dependence on sleep medications, leading to long-term use of hypnotics. Over time, dependence on hypnotics can lead to problems with memory deficits and nocturnal falls among older adults. If insomnia remains untreated, it can exacerbate psychiatric conditions. Studies examining the temporal relationship between insomnia and depression have found that the occurrence of insomnia symptoms tends to precede the occurrence of depression (Johnson, Roth, & Breslau, 2006; Ohayon & Roth, 2003), thereby indicating that insomnia is a risk factor in the development of depression (Johnson et al., 2006).

Beyond the consequences for the individual, insomnia has significant occupational and economic consequences. It is associated with an elevated risk of both working and nonworking injuries (Kessler et al., 2012). In the workplace, insomnia-related absenteeism has been estimated to have an annual indirect cost of $970.6 million, and insomnia-related productivity losses are estimated at $5 billion (Daley, Morin, LeBlanc, Grégoire, & Savard, 2009). The significant consequences of insomnia clearly indicate a need to find effective treatments for this condition.

Etiology of Insomnia

CAUSES OF SLEEP DISTURBANCE

What are the causes of insomnia? Recognizing the conceptual distinction between acute sleep disturbance and an insomnia disorder is important in answering this question. First, there are many causes of acute sleep disturbance on any given night. Some of these factors include the use of wake-promoting substances (e.g., caffeine), daytime napping, exposure to bright light at night, or sleeping past the normal wake-up time. These can lead to disturbances in the two systems that regulate sleep physiology (see Figure 1.2). Together, these two systems interact to promote an intrinsic drive and rhythm for sleep and wakefulness that is called the *two-process model of sleep regulation* (Borbély, 1982; Borbély & Achermann, 1999).

The first process in the model is the homeostatic drive for sleep, also known as *Process S*, which regulates a "sleep appetite" that accumulates across the wake episode. This system creates pressure for sleep to occur on the basis of the amount of time awake. It is generally a linear process, such that the longer the amount of time awake, the greater the sleep pressure. Therefore, behaviors such as taking a nap in the evening can reduce the pressure to sleep at bedtime, creating difficulty falling asleep. This concept is similar to the notion that having a snack shortly before a meal will spoil the appetite for food. As part of Process S, adenosine, an inhibitory neurotransmitter found in the central nervous system, accumulates across wakefulness and is associated with sleepiness. Caffeine is an adenosine antagonist, blocking the action of the neurotransmitter. Therefore, drinking caffeine has the effect of blocking the accumulation of sleepiness, thus allowing an individual to be alert, even after many

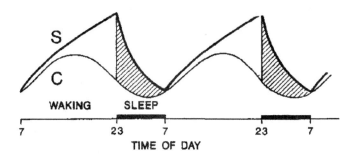

FIGURE 1.2

Two-process model of sleep regulation. Process S (sleep homeostasis) reflects the accumulation of sleepiness across waking episodes, which subsequently dissipates during the sleep phase. Process C (circadian process) regulates the timing of alertness and sleep, interacting with Process S to regulate phases of sleep and wakefulness. From "A Two Process Model of Sleep Regulation," by A. A. Borbély, 1982, *Human Neurobiology*, 1, p. 198. Copyright 1982 by Springer. Adapted with permission.

hours of being awake. This is why drinking caffeine too close to bedtime can create difficulty falling asleep.

The second system is the circadian system, or *Process C*, which is an endogenous system that regulates the timing of alertness and sleep by generating alerting signals and creating a daily rhythm known as a *circadian rhythm*. Unlike Process S, Process C is independent of sleeping and waking states and primarily generates alerting signals, rather than sleepy signals. Process C is sensitive to light–dark cycles in the environment, particularly at night and in the morning. At night, when darkness is predominant, Process C regulates the release of melatonin, which serves as a cue for the brain to turn off its wake-promoting regions and prepare for sleep. For most individuals, melatonin is released about 1 to 2 hours before the regular bedtime. Therefore, exposure to bright light around this time of night can suppress the release of melatonin, resulting in the wake-promoting regions of the brain to remain active. As a result, it might be difficult to disengage from waking activities, which can create difficulty falling asleep. In the morning, Process C is very sensitive to light exposure near the wake-up time, which helps to reset the circadian rhythm for the day. Keeping a regular wake-up time throughout the weekday and weekend is one of the most important factors for strengthening the consistency of the circadian rhythm. In fact, a regular wake-up time is biologically more important than a regular bedtime because the timing of Process C is more closely synchronized with the wake-up time. Dysregulation in Process C is often a biological factor that distinguishes insomnia phenotypes such that a delay in the timing of Process C is associated with trouble falling asleep, whereas advanced timing of Process C is associated with early morning awakenings.

In extreme cases, misalignment of Process C with the desired sleep phase can lead to circadian rhythm sleep–wake disorders. This category of sleep disorders includes delayed sleep-phase disorder and advanced sleep-phase disorder. In delayed sleep-phase disorder, the endogenous circadian rhythm is delayed relative to the individual's behavioral sleep–wake patterns, leading to prolonged difficulty falling asleep and difficulty waking up early in the morning, with little or no difficulty maintaining sleep. This is common in adolescents and young adults who are "night owls," whereas Process C shifts to a later time. In advanced sleep-phase disorder, the endogenous circadian sleep phase occurs at a relatively early time in the evening. As a result, these individuals fall asleep easily but wake up earlier than desired and have difficulty staying asleep until the desired wake-up time. This is common in older adults who are "morning larks," as there is a shift in Process C toward an earlier time. Individuals with delayed sleep-phase and advance sleep-phase disorders might present with complaints of insomnia symptoms, but these individuals usually do not experience the same level of distress about their sleep. Furthermore, realigning the circadian sleep phase with their behavioral sleep patterns typically resolves the sleep disturbance and daytime complaints. Longitudinal assessment using sleep diaries over 1 to 2 weeks can help discern a circadian rhythm sleep–wake disorder from an insomnia disorder (see the section on conducting pre-MBTI assessments in Chapter 4).

Most people with insomnia do not realize the impact that their behaviors have on these two systems of sleep regulation. For example, taking naps in the late afternoon or evening might reduce sleepiness and temporarily improves functioning, but it can deplete the pressure for sleep in Process S. Spending more time in bed might seem like a reasonable way to make up for sleep loss, but it also reduces the amount of time we are awake to generate a sleep appetite. Although it might seem counterintuitive to those with insomnia, Process S is actually optimized the longer we are awake and out of bed. In other words, the longer the period of continuous wakefulness, the more likely we are to have consolidated sleep. Similarly, people with insomnia often sleep past their regular wake-up time as a means of compensating for a poor night of sleep or to "catch up" on sleep during the weekends. However, doing so can disrupt the circadian rhythm, leading to difficulty sleeping or feeling alert, respectively, at the appropriate time of day. In fact, people who constantly delay their sleep patterns by several hours over the weekend because of social obligations (e.g., staying out late) create a dysregulation in Process C that has become known as *social jet lag* because it mimics the effects of traveling across several time zones. The two-factor model of sleep regulation provides a background for some of the activities and discussions that are presented as part of MBTI in Part II of this volume.

In addition to dysregulation of the sleep systems, there are times when acute stress, such as an argument with a family member or an urgent deadline, causes sleep disturbance. In these situations, the brain responds to the perceived stress by activating the sympathetic nervous system (SNS), also known as *the fight-or-flight system*. Activation of the SNS can serve to override the regulation of sleep physiology as described in the preceding text. Although it can be very obvious at times—as in a rush of adrenaline—in modern society, activation of the SNS is more likely to be at a low to moderate level and not always consciously detectable. Thus, when we have an argument with a family member, our body can be in a state of elevated activation, or *hyperarousal*, which creates sleep disturbance.

Several studies have found that compared with good sleepers, people with insomnia have several physiological signs that are consistent with a state of hyperarousal, including elevations in 24-hour metabolic rate (Bonnet & Arand, 1995), higher daytime body temperature (Adam, Tomeny, & Oswald, 1986), more low-frequency heart rate variability during sleep (Bonnet & Arand, 1998), and higher 24-hour cortisol secretion (Vgontzas et al., 1998). There is also evidence of increased mental activity, or *cognitive hyperarousal*. Studies have found that people with insomnia report higher levels of presleep cognitive activity (Nicassio, Mendlowitz, Fussell, & Petras, 1985) and tend to have sleep-related cognitions of a more negative tone (Kuisk, Bertelson, & Walsh, 1989) compared with those of normal sleepers. People with insomnia also report more unhelpful beliefs and attitudes about sleep (Carney & Edinger, 2006; Morin, Stone, Trinkle, Mercer, & Remsberg, 1993), demonstrating a more rigid or catastrophic view of sleep that increases anxiety and cognitive arousal. For people with insomnia who completed a behavioral treatment for insomnia, those who had at least one insomnia episode (at least 4 consecutive weeks with insomnia symptoms) during the follow-up period had higher presleep arousal and sleep effort at the end of treatment compared with those with no insomnia episodes during follow-up (Ong, Shapiro, & Manber, 2009). Collectively, these studies serve to demonstrate that cognitive and physiological arousal play important etiological roles in sleep disturbance associated with insomnia.

At the organism level, the physiological states generated by the SNS and the sleep systems can provide an indication of the activation and deactivation of these systems. Attending to these states can guide behavioral responses, such as when to go to bed or when to engage in relaxing activities. The two most relevant states are sleepiness and fatigue.

Sleepiness is defined as the propensity to fall asleep and represents a physiological need for sleep. It can be self-reported through questionnaires or rating scales, and it can be measured objectively (Shen, Barbera, & Shapiro, 2006). Self-reported descriptions of sleepiness include drowsiness, fighting to stay awake, or falling asleep unintentionally. In sleep laboratories, the Multiple Sleep Latency Test (MSLT; Carskadon et al., 1986) is used as an objective measure of daytime sleepiness. The MSLT involves a series of five naps that are spaced 2 hours apart and is conducted under controlled conditions in which the patient is not otherwise allowed to sleep or consume substances that can affect sleep or wakefulness. Abnormal sleepiness is typically defined by averaging less than 8 minutes to fall asleep across each nap. Sleepiness is most closely associated with the accumulation of sleep drive in Process S, as described in the preceding text.

Fatigue is another state that is often used interchangeably with sleepiness in colloquial language but has a very specific meaning in sleep medicine. In this context, *fatigue* is a complex construct that involves an interpretation of the mental and physical energy available or the degree to which it takes energy to engage in an activity. There are no objective measures or tests for fatigue, but there are self-reported measures, which include items such as lack of energy, a feeling of lethargy, decreased strength, or diminished ability to engage in activities. Notably, fatigue is not highly correlated with the ability to fall asleep quickly because it involves activation of the sleep systems and the SNS. Although there might be a high sleep drive from Process S, there is also hyperarousal from the SNS, which prevents falling asleep quickly. As a result, those with insomnia frequently describe a state of being "tired but wired" in which sleep is strongly desired but is not likely to happen because of SNS activation.

Individuals with insomnia often confuse the state of fatigue with sleepiness. They often decide to go to bed when they feel fatigued but are not actually sleepy; in other words, they have low energy or no desire to engage in activities, but when given the opportunity to sleep there is not a sufficient biological drive for sleepiness. A study using the MSLT found that individuals with insomnia took longer to fall asleep across the daytime naps compared with control participants (Stepanski, Zorick, Roehrs, Young, & Roth, 1988). Thus, these individuals with insomnia were less sleepy than were healthy control participants during the daytime. Furthermore, it has been recommended that excessive sleepiness be removed as a criterion for insomnia disorders because there is little evidence that people with insomnia are excessively sleepy during the day (Singareddy, Bixler, & Vgontzas, 2010). The importance of discerning the difference between sleepiness and fatigue is discussed in Chapter 6.

BEYOND SLEEP DISTURBANCE: ETIOLOGY OF CHRONIC INSOMNIA

The causes of sleep disturbance provide an understanding of what might trigger or precipitate the onset of an insomnia disorder. However, this is only part of the story. According to the current diagnostic nosologies (e.g., American Academy of Sleep Medicine, 2014; American Psychiatric Association, 2013), recall that an insomnia disorder includes sleep-specific symptoms plus significant waking distress or impairment despite adequate opportunity to sleep. Therefore, an insomnia disorder is a 24-hour problem, not just a problem that occurs at night. Furthermore, the associated waking distress includes cognitions, behaviors, and physiological changes that develop over time. Several etiological models have been proposed to explain how these factors are involved in the development and maintenance of chronic insomnia.

The biobehavioral model, also known as the 3-P model, is arguably the most influential and widely accepted etiological model of chronic insomnia (see Figure 1.3). Spielman, Caruso, and Glovinsky (1987) proposed three factors that are involved in the development and maintenance of insomnia. First, certain *predisposing factors* serve as a diathesis, which can increase the overall likelihood that an individual will develop sleep disturbance at any given time. These predisposing factors include extreme circadian preferences (i.e., morning vs. evening type), biological predispositions toward hyperarousal, or psychological traits related to anxiety and depression. When a predisposing factor interacts with a *precipitating factor*, or triggering event, typically in the form of a psychological or biological stress, the result is acute sleep disturbance. As discussed earlier, sleep disturbance can be considered a natural stress response, and for many individuals, sleep quantity and quality improve once the precipitating factor or stress has abated. However, some individuals begin to engage in behavioral changes in response to the acute sleep disturbance, such as extending time in bed by getting into bed earlier, sleeping later in the morning, or taking naps during the day. Some might also begin taking sleep medication at night and consuming caffeine during the day in an effort to regulate sleep and wakefulness. Although these responses might seem logical, the changes inadvertently maintain the insomnia disorder and are thus considered *perpetuating factors*, which can reduce the sleep drive (e.g., extending time in bed) or create circadian misalignment (e.g., sleeping late and varying wake-up time). In addition to changes in sleep-related behaviors, perpetuating factors can include changes in sleep-related cognitions. Many people with insomnia become anxious and frustrated about their inability to sleep. Some begin to worry about the effects of sleep loss on work performance or daytime functioning. Frequently, these thoughts lead to increased effort to "solve the problem

FIGURE 1.3

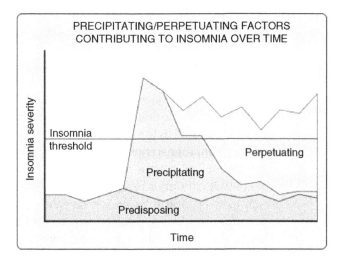

The 3-P model of insomnia. The biobehavioral model posits that the development and maintenance of chronic insomnia disorders involve an interaction between predisposing, precipitating, and perpetuating factors. From *Principles and Practice of Sleep Medicine* (5th ed., p. 843), by M. H. Kryger, T. Roth, and W. C. Dement (Eds.), 2011, Philadelphia, PA: Elsevier. Copyright 2011 by Elsevier. Adapted with permission.

of not sleeping," which creates distress about sleep, thus maintaining a 24-hour problem that is now a chronic insomnia disorder. According to this model, chronic insomnia disorder is a combination of predisposing, precipitating, and perpetuating factors. Furthermore, this model shows how the reactions to sleep disturbance can play a crucial etiological role in creating waking distress.

Subsequent models have built on the foundation of the 3-P model. Perlis, Giles, Mendelson, Bootzin, and Wyatt (1997) proposed a neurocognitive model of insomnia that focuses on cortical changes that occur with the perpetuating factors. These changes include those in sensory processing, information processing, and long-term memory formation that lead to alterations in the perception of the sleep experience. For example, comparisons of self-reports and objectively measured sleep–wakefulness data show that individuals with insomnia often overestimate wakefulness and underestimate sleep. Studies examining the microarchitecture of sleep in people with insomnia have found evidence of elevated beta-electroencephalogram (EEG) activity during non–rapid eye movement (REM) sleep (Merica, Blois, & Gaillard, 1998). Beta-EEG activity is typically associated with consciousness and could explain why people with insomnia sometimes report "light sleep" or "not sleeping at all," despite polysomnography recordings demonstrating that the person was indeed sleeping.

Espie (2002) proposed a psychobiological inhibition model with a different conceptualization of the hyperarousal in the context of insomnia. Rather than a constant elevation of arousal, as proposed by others, Espie posited that people with insomnia might have difficulty with dearousal at night. According to the psychobiological model, good sleepers are able to dearouse appropriately at night when appropriate biological and environmental cues are present and do not put effort into falling asleep. However, people with insomnia react to sleep disturbance by putting selective attention to sleep, and they do not recognize the same cues for sleep and wakefulness, thereby increasing the effort and intention to sleep. As a result, they are unable to dearouse, both cognitively and physiologically. Evidence to support this model comes from a study that used positron emission tomography to assess cerebral glucose metabolism in patients with insomnia compared with that of healthy participants while awake and during non-REM sleep (Nofzinger et al., 2004). Patients with insomnia showed a smaller decline in metabolic rate in wake-promoting regions of the brain during the transition from wakefulness to the first 20 minutes of sleep. This evidence supports the concept that in these individuals with insomnia, there was a failure to "turn off" wake promoting systems in the brain, or de-arouse appropriately during the transition from a waking state to a sleeping state.

Morin and colleagues (1993) proposed a cognitive behavioral model that adds cognitions as a perpetuating factor in chronic insomnia. Describing insomnia as a cycle, Morin et al.'s (1993) model features cognitive and emotional components that include maladaptive beliefs and attitudes about sleep that develop with persistent sleep disturbance, such as worrying about sleep, frustration over the consequences of not sleeping, and unrealistic or rigid expectations about sleep (e.g., must get 8 hours of sleep). These unhelpful cognitions then interact with maladaptive habits (e.g., excessive time in bed, napping, irregular sleep schedule), the true consequences of insufficient sleep (e.g., fatigue, mood disturbances, performance impairments), and elevated arousal to create a vicious cycle of insomnia. Building on Morin and colleagues' (1993) model, Harvey (2002) proposed a cognitive model of insomnia by focusing exclusively on the role of cognitive processes that occur during the nighttime and daytime. This model applies many theories of anxiety, including worry, selective attention monitoring, misperception of sleep, unhelpful beliefs, and safety behaviors in the context of insomnia. It is interesting to note that the model also suggests that these processes can occur with or without real deficits in sleep and daytime functioning.

In summary, understanding the etiology of insomnia requires recognition of the differences between acute sleep disturbance and a chronic insomnia disorder. The causes of acute sleep disturbance are difficult to predict and generally involve disturbances in sleep physiology, activation of the SNS, or both. When these sleep disturbances persist, engagement in maladaptive cognitive and behavioral changes in response to the acute sleep disturbance transforms the acute sleep disturbance into a chronic insomnia disorder, a 24-hour problem that includes waking distress in addition to the nighttime sleep disturbance. Hyperarousal in the form of elevated arousal or a failure to dearouse is prominent in the state of chronic insomnia. These concepts play an important role in understanding the approach for using mindfulness meditation as an intervention for insomnia, as is discussed in Part II of this volume.

Current Treatments for Insomnia

2

T here are currently many different approaches to treating insomnia disorders, and they have varying levels of scientific evidence to support them. These approaches can be grouped into the following three categories: (a) *pharmacological*, (b) *nonpharmacological*, and (c) *complementary, alternative, and integrative*.

First, pharmacological treatments, including prescription medications and over-the-counter (OTC) drugs, are reviewed. The main benefit of these treatments is the immediate impact on reducing sleep disturbance, but issues of drug dependence and side effects mitigate the overall benefit-to-risk profile.

Next, nonpharmacological treatments are reviewed. These include behavioral and cognitive techniques that are typically delivered by a behavioral specialist. These treatments can be customized to patient needs, and the benefits of treatment are sustained beyond the end of treatment. However, they do not have the immediate impact of prescription medications, and there are limitations in the number of practitioners who are qualified to deliver these treatments.

http://dx.doi.org/10.1037/14952-003

Mindfulness-Based Therapy for Insomnia, by J. C. Ong

Finally, complementary and integrative approaches include natural products, body-based interventions, and mind–body interventions. These are commonly adopted by people who prefer a "natural" or "healthy" way of living. However, scientific evidence regarding efficacy is generally of poor quality; thus, the clinical value of these treatments is unclear. Because patients often have questions about the costs and benefits of various treatments for insomnia, mindfulness-based therapy for insomnia (MBTI) instructors should be positioned to help them make informed decisions about treatment options.

Pharmacological Treatments for Insomnia

The idea of taking a sleeping pill, or a hypnotic, to facilitate sleep seems like a simple concept, but the wide variety of substances that have been used to help people fall asleep belies this. This section provides an overview of the evidence for pharmacological treatments, including prescription medications, nonprescription medications (i.e., OTC medications), and alcohol. Table 2.1 provides a summary of the pharmacological treatments for insomnia.

The neurotransmitter gamma-aminobutyric acid (GABA) is an inhibitory neurotransmitter within the central nervous system that is involved in sedation. Therefore, drugs that act as GABA agonists have been used to facilitate sleep. These include the traditional benzodiazepines, such as clonazepam, lorazepam, temazepam, and triazolam, as well as the newer nonbenzodiazepines, including zolpidem, eszopiclone, and zaleplon. These nonbenzodiazepines, often referred to as *z-drugs* because of their names, also act as GABA agonists but are structurally different from benzodiazepines. Both benzodiazepines and z-drugs can decrease sleep onset latency (SOL) and increase total sleep time (TST) with moderate to large effect sizes. A meta-analysis on benzodiazepines found that with only 1 to 7 days of use, TST increased by about 62 minutes, and sleep onset was reduced by about 4 minutes when measured objectively (Holbrook, Crowther, Lotter, Cheng, & King, 2000). Another meta-analysis examining both benzodiazepines and two z-drugs (zolpidem and zopiclone) found that these drugs increased TST about 40 minutes and decreased sleep latency by about 14 minutes (Smith et al., 2002). A large-scale study comparing eszopiclone to placebo found an increase of 70 minutes in TST and a reduction of 42 minutes on sleep onset for patients using eszopiclone for 1 week (Krystal et al., 2003). These findings indicate that both benzodiazepines and z-drugs are effective at increasing TST and reducing

TABLE 2.1

Common Pharmacological Treatments for Insomnia (Hypnotic Medications)

Generic name	Trade name	Class	Mechanism of action	Duration of action
Flurazepam	Dalmane	Benzodiazepine	$GABA_A$ agonist	Long
Clonazepam	Klonopin	Benzodiazepine	$GABA_A$ agonist	Long
Quazepam	Doral	Benzodiazepine	$GABA_A$ agonist	Long
Diazepam	Valium	Benzodiazepine	$GABA_A$ agonist	Long
Estazolam	ProSom	Benzodiazepine	$GABA_A$ agonist	Intermediate
Lorazepam	Ativan	Benzodiazepine	$GABA_A$ agonist	Intermediate
Alprazolam	Xanax	Benzodiazepine	$GABA_A$ agonist	Intermediate
Temazepam	Restoril	Benzodiazepine	$GABA_A$ agonist	Intermediate
Triazolam	Halcion	Benzodiazepine	$GABA_A$ agonist	Short
Zolpidem	Ambien	Non-benzodiazepine	$GABA_A$ agonist	Short
Zaleplon	Sonata	Non-benzodiazepine	$GABA_A$ agonist	Short
Eszopiclone	Lunesta	Non-benzodiazepine	$GABA_A$ agonist	Short
Diphenhydramine	Benadryl	Antihistamine	H_1 antagonist	Short
Ramelteon	Rozerem	Melatonin agonist	MT_1 and MT_2 agonist	Short
Suvorexant	Belsomra	Orexin antagonist	OX_1 and OX_2 antagonist	Short

Note. GABA = gamma-aminobutyric acid; H = histamine; MT = melatonin; OX = orexin.

SOL. Furthermore, these effects occur relatively quickly, within the first week of use.

When evaluating the benefits of these sleep medications, their side effects need to be considered. One of the drawbacks of using benzodiazepines and z-drugs is residual drowsiness or grogginess in the morning. As a result, some patients have difficulty getting out of bed or have impaired cognitive or motor skills in the morning. This is more prominent in longer acting benzodiazepines, such as flurazepam and clonazepam, and less common in short-acting benzodiazepines and z-drugs. Also, taking medication in the middle of the night or not spending sufficient time in bed can increase the risk of these side effects. Amnestic episodes are another common side effect that has been reported with benzodiazepines and z-drugs. These amnestic episodes include behaviors or activities that individuals engage in after taking the medication and of which they have no memory the next day. Reports of amnestic episodes include eating behaviors, talking on the phone, and operating motor vehicles. These issues have raised concerns about the widespread use of these medications for sleep.

A second class of drugs that are used as hypnotics are melatonin agonists. Melatonin is a hormone that is released by the pineal gland and regulates the timing of the circadian clock (Process C). Given that an etiological factor for some individuals with insomnia is dysregulation of the circadian rhythm, melatonin agonists help to align the body's internal clock with the desired sleep period. In a study of over 400 adults, ramelteon was found to decrease sleep latency and increase TST compared with placebo (Zammit et al., 2007). One key advantage with ramelteon is the general lack of dependence or abuse associated with the drug. Reported side effects of ramelteon include residual daytime sleepiness, dizziness, nausea, and in rare cases, anaphylactic reactions and suicide in people with a preexisting depression. This is the only melatonin agonist that has been approved by the U.S. Food and Drug Administration for long-term treatment of insomnia.

The most recent class of medications to receive approval as a hypnotic is the orexin antagonist. Orexin, also called hypocretin, is a neurotransmitter that is involved in the regulation of arousal, wakefulness, and appetite. In the context of sleep disorders, orexin deficiency has been implicated in the etiology of narcolepsy (Nishino, Ripley, Overeem, Lammers, & Mignot, 2000), where a failure to maintain wakefulness or cortical arousal leads to excessive daytime sleepiness and sleep attacks. An orexin antagonist called suvorexant was developed that blocks the action of orexin and causes sleepiness. A double-blind, clinical trial testing suvorexant on people with insomnia found that suvorexant decreased SOL and improved sleep efficiency (Herring et al., 2012). In August 2014, suvorexant was approved by the U.S. Food and Drug Administration (FDA) for the treatment of insomnia. Because it has been approved only recently, there are no long-term data available or any comparative studies with other benzodiazepines, z-drugs, or melatonin agonists.

In addition to these hypnotic medications, several medications classified as antidepressants or antipsychotics have been used as an off-label treatment for insomnia. Common antidepressants used for insomnia include amitriptyline, doxepin, trazodone, and mirtazapine. Although these drugs are frequently prescribed by psychiatrists, the evidence base for efficacy and adverse events is rather scant compared with that for the previously reviewed medications. Atypical antipsychotics, such as quetiapine, have also been used for treating insomnia. Much like antidepressants, there is little specific evidence on this use of antipsychotics.

Beyond these prescription medications, there are nonprescription drugs and substances that are used as self-medication for insomnia. Patients often use these as a first step before seeking professional evaluation, or they use them in combination with a prescribed medication. OTC medications that have diphenhydramine as the primary active ingredient are the most common nonprescription medications for insomnia. Diphenhydramine is an antihistamine that can produce sleepiness as a side effect. However, there is little evidence to support efficacy or to document adverse events when it is used to treat insomnia. Alcohol is another substance that is commonly used informally by patients to help promote sleep. Although alcohol can have sedating effects, it has very disruptive effects on sleep architecture. Specifically, alcohol is a potent suppressor of REM (rapid eye movement) sleep and to a lesser extent can suppress slow wave sleep, two of the most important stages of sleep. Furthermore, alcohol can suppress respiration, which can exacerbate sleep-disordered breathing (e.g., sleep apnea), which frequently co-occurs with insomnia.

The American Academy of Sleep Medicine (AASM) has provided guidelines on the use of pharmacological treatments for insomnia (Schutte-Rodin, Broch, Buysse, Dorsey, & Sateia, 2008). The choice of medication should be directed by clinical indications and patient-centered considerations (e.g., patient preferences, goals, costs). Regarding the order of treatment, the recommended first-line treatment is a short- to intermediate-acting benzodiazepine, z-drug, or ramelteon. Subsequently, sedating antidepressants should be considered, followed by a combination of the first-line treatment with an antidepressant. Notably, the AASM recommended short-term hypnotic treatments for most patients, with long-term use reserved for people with chronic comorbid illnesses, severe insomnia, or for patients who do not respond to other treatments (i.e., refractory insomnia). Drug dependence and drug tolerance are potential factors that raise concerns about the long-term use of sleep medications. In the case of insomnia, psychological dependence occurs when use of the drug continues because of a belief that the medication is needed to sleep. It is very common for people with insomnia to experience a phenomenon known as *rebound insomnia,* which is a brief worsening of sleep on abrupt discontinuation of hypnotic medication use. Typically, rebound insomnia lasts only 1 or 2 nights during which sleep is worse relative to baseline and is more prominent in medications with a short or intermediate half-life. Unfortunately, people who experience rebound insomnia are reinforced to believe that they need the medication to sleep. Drug tolerance occurs when there is a diminished response to the drug after repeated exposure. In the context of insomnia, tolerance might lead to dose escalation at the beginning of the night or taking additional doses in the middle of the night. The latter situation not only increases the dose but also raises concerns about next-day functioning. Both of these situations could increase the risk of experiencing side effects and should be avoided.

In general, FDA-approved medications for insomnia can be effective for reducing nocturnal symptoms, and these effects are seen within the first days of use. However, these benefits need to be weighed against the potential risks of side effects, drug dependency, and drug tolerance. Much like the other treatments, sleep medication is a viable tool that can be helpful for many patients, especially those experiencing transient or acute insomnia. However, long-term use of sleep medication should be carefully managed by an experienced physician, and consideration should be given to a nonpharmacological approach either as an adjunct or an eventual substitute for sleep medication.

Nonpharmacological Treatments for Insomnia

Nonpharmacological treatments for insomnia have largely been developed by merging the findings on sleep physiology in basic sleep science with behavioral and cognitive theories in applied psychological science. Over the past 4 decades, these treatments have evolved from single-modality treatments to multicomponent ones in a manner that parallels the evolution of cognitive behavior therapy at a broad level. Behavioral treatments for insomnia began with strategies grounded in behavioral principles. As discussed in Chapter 1, the conceptualization of insomnia focused on the notion that sleep disruptions are caused by elevated arousal. As a result, early attempts to treat insomnia involved relaxation strategies, such as progressive muscle relaxation (Jacobson, 1938) and biofeedback (Hauri, 1981), which were aimed at reducing physiological arousal stemming from the sympathetic nervous system. Bootzin (1972), one of the most influential psychologists who studied sleep and insomnia, applied the concepts of stimulus control to the treatment of insomnia, proposing that repeated pairing of the bed with an inability to sleep leads to the bed becoming a stimulus for conditioned arousal. To break this association and reestablish the bed as a place for sleep, individuals with insomnia are provided with a set of instructions, called *stimulus control*, advising them to leave the bed when they are unable to sleep and to go to bed (or return to bed in the middle of the night) only when sleepy. In addition, the individual is asked to avoid doing other waking activities in bed (e.g., no television, no reading) and to wake up at the same time each morning, regardless of the amount of sleep. Over time, these instructions result in strengthening the bed as a stimulus for sleep, thus creating a greater likelihood of reducing arousal, falling asleep, and staying asleep. Spielman, Saskin, and Thorpy (1987) developed *sleep restriction therapy*, a behavioral treatment restricting time in bed to mobilize the homeostatic drive to sleep and prevent compensation for poor sleep by spending extra time in bed. First, patients are instructed to limit the time in bed to match the amount of sleep they are currently receiving. For example, if they report sleeping only 6 hours each night, time in bed is limited to a fixed 6-hour window. Gradually, time in bed is systematically expanded as the patient experiences less total wake time and higher sleep efficiency, an index of the percentage of time asleep divided by the time in bed. Another influential set of instructions known as *sleep hygiene* was introduced by Hauri (1977). Sleep hygiene consisted of instructions for modifying behaviors and activities related to sleep, such as not exercising late at night, avoiding caffeine and alcohol close to bedtime, and avoiding naps during the daytime. These instructions were informed by research on environmental and behavioral factors that were found to have a negative impact on sleep.

Unfortunately, the term *sleep hygiene* has taken on a more generalized meaning and is often misused. Instead of the initial instructions that Hauri recommended, many people now use the term *sleep hygiene* to refer to a broad range of behavioral recommendations, including elements of sleep restriction and stimulus control. However, each behavioral treatment has its distinct theory, logic, and delivery, and lumping these treatments into a broad category of sleep hygiene creates confusion for patients and health care providers. Furthermore, the original sleep hygiene instructions have been found to yield only small effect sizes, and it is not considered to be an effective treatment for insomnia (Stepanski & Wyatt, 2003). Careful use of the term *sleep hygiene* and recognition that it does not include stimulus control and sleep restriction is needed.

Morin, Stone, Trinkle, Mercer, and Remsberg (1993) led the development of cognitive behavior therapy for insomnia (CBT-I), which combined the single-modality behavioral treatments with cognitive therapy to form a multitreatment package. They found that people with insomnia hold maladaptive beliefs and attitudes about sleep. Consequently, they adapted techniques from Beck and colleagues' (Beck, Rush, Shaw, & Emery, 1979) *Cognitive Therapy of Depression* to target these maladaptive sleep-related cognitions. These techniques focused on catastrophizing and probability overestimation, two cognitive errors that were common among individuals with insomnia (Morin, 1993). For example, some people with insomnia hold onto the belief that if they do not achieve the desired amount of sleep, they will not be able to function the next day. Although it is true that sleep deprivation can impact next-day functioning, it is also possible to perform at an adequate level. In this scenario, cognitive techniques can help patients restructure rigid beliefs by asking them to consider the belief as a hypothesis and to collect evidence to test the hypothesis. This unveils a range of probability rather than definitive outcomes. Cognitive techniques, such as this one, are then combined with stimulus control, sleep restriction, and sleep hygiene into an 8-week therapy that is known today as CBT-I. An important advantage of CBT-I is that it is possible to customize the various treatment components to meet the specific needs of each individual patient. See Table 2.2 for a summary of nonpharmacological treatments.

There is a substantial evidence base to support the efficacy of behavioral treatment packages, including CBT-I and multicomponent behavior therapies without cognitive therapy. Randomized clinical trials have reported moderate to large effect sizes on sleep parameters, with about 26% to 43% of patients achieving full remission from insomnia when categorically

TABLE 2.2

Nonpharmacological Treatments for Insomnia

Treatment	Description
Relaxation training	Relaxation exercises to reduce physiological and cognitive arousal
Stimulus control	Set of instructions for bedroom-related behaviors designed to reestablish the bed as a stimulus for sleep
Sleep restriction	Sleep schedule used to reduce time in bed to increase homeostatic sleep drive, thereby improving sleep efficiency
Sleep hygiene	Set of instructions to eliminate habits that are counterproductive for sleep
Cognitive therapy	Therapeutic techniques to address maladaptive thoughts and beliefs that interfere with sleep and daytime functioning
Multicomponent behavior therapy	Treatment package consisting of stimulus control and sleep restriction (core) with the option of relaxation training and sleep hygiene—cognitive therapy is not included
Cognitive behavior therapy for insomnia (CBT-I)	Treatment package consisting of stimulus control, sleep restriction, and cognitive therapy (core), with the option of relaxation training and sleep hygiene

defined criteria are applied (Buysse et al., 2011; Edinger, Wohlgemuth, Radtke, Marsh, & Quillian, 2001; Epstein, Sidani, Bootzin, & Belyea, 2012; Jacobs, Pace-Schott, Stickgold, & Otto, 2004; Morin, Colecchi, Stone, Sood, & Brink, 1999; Sivertsen et al., 2006). When compared with medications, CBT-I appears to have more durable effects (Morin et al., 1999). Meta-analyses and reviews have found that about 70% to 80% of patients benefit from CBT-I with reductions in SOL and the amount of wake time after sleep onset by about 50% and a more modest increase in TST from 6.0 to 6.5 hours (Morin, Bastien, & Savard, 2003). Currently, the AASM practice guidelines list CBT-I and multicomponent behavior therapy without cognitive therapy as the first-line nonpharmacological treatment of choice (Morgenthaler et al., 2006; Schutte-Rodin et al., 2008).

As with other forms of psychotherapy, there are few known side effects of these behavioral treatment packages. One potential side effect is daytime sleepiness, which is most commonly associated with sleep restriction therapy (Kyle, Morgan, Spiegelhalder, & Espie, 2011). Given that sleep restriction involves reducing time in bed, some sleep deprivation might occur that could exacerbate daytime sleepiness. Compared with medications, the benefits of CBT-I are slower to emerge. Whereas medications tend to be effective within 1 week, the full benefits of CBT-I do not emerge until 4 to 8 weeks after initiation of treatment. As a psychological treatment, it requires time and effort to attend clinic visits and also to implement the treatment recommendations at home in between treatment sessions. Some patients are not able to devote sufficient time and energy to this process and, thus, are not able to achieve the full benefits of this treatment approach. Finally, an important limitation is the number of qualified practitioners to deliver CBT-I. There are currently about 250 practitioners who are board certified in behavioral sleep medicine. Patients who live in rural areas or more remote locations often do not have access to a practitioner who has training in delivering CBT-I; therefore, given the prevalence of insomnia, the supply is not meeting the demand.

In the early 21st century, behavioral sleep medicine (BSM) emerged as a distinct specialty within psychology and behavioral medicine. Involving psychologists, physicians, and nurses, this multidisciplinary area was organized to help improve the delivery of behavioral services, promote behavioral and psychological research related to sleep, and to regulate the training of BSM practitioners. In 2010, the Society of Behavioral Sleep Medicine (SBSM) was formed following the Ponte Vedra consensus conference (D. J. Taylor, Perlis, McCrae, & Smith, 2010). Since that time, the SBSM has been working to further establish and validate the role of psychologists in sleep. In 2013, the American Psychological Association approved sleep psychology as a formal specialty, and further efforts are underway by the SBSM to apply for a specialty examination with the American Board of Professional Psychology.

Complementary, Alternative, and Integrative Medicine

Many people use complementary and alternative medicine (CAM), also known as integrative medicine, for insomnia. In the case of insomnia, these treatments might be an alternative to the traditional treatments or in addition to the first-line treatments described earlier. CAM treatments for insomnia consist of a diverse group of interventions and techniques including natural products, body-based (or manipulative) interventions, and mind–body interventions. In 2002, over 1.6 million Americans were using a CAM treatment for insomnia symptoms (Pearson, Johnson, & Nahin, 2006). In 2007, 45% of adults with insomnia symptoms were using CAM annually (Bertisch, Wells, Smith, & McCarthy, 2012). See Table 2.3 for a summary of complementary, alternative, and integrative medicine approaches to insomnia.

Use of natural products for sleep is high, particularly for young women with a high level of education (Pearson et al., 2006). The most common natural products used for insomnia are chamomile, valerian, St. John's wort, and kava kava. Although there is a general perception

TABLE 2.3

Complementary, Alternative, and Integrative Treatments for Insomnia

Class	Treatment/technique	Comment
Natural products	Chamomile Valerian St. John's wort Kava kava	Herbal remedies or natural products that can be purchased over the counter; limited evidence of efficacy and some safety concerns
Body-based interventions	Acupuncture Massage	Evidence for acupuncture is unclear because of poor quality of studies. No randomized controlled studies on massage.
Mind–body interventions	Meditation Yoga Tai chi	Approaches that are aimed at self-regulating the mind and body; evidence is promising for insomnia

that use of natural products reflects a healthy lifestyle, research has yielded very little evidence to support the health benefits of natural products in the case of insomnia, and there are some indications of potential risk. Furthermore, in many countries, these products are not subjected to the regulations associated with prescription medications, which raises questions about the purity of the substance.

Body-based therapies focus on bodily systems and involve structural manipulation of specific points, such as bones, joints, soft tissue, or circulation. Acupuncture and massage are the two most common body-based therapies that are used to treat insomnia. Several systematic reviews on acupuncture for insomnia have been conducted and concluded that acupuncture with manual needle stimulation based in traditional Chinese medicine was significantly more effective than sleep hygiene treatment and sham acupuncture and of equivalent or superior efficacy to benzodiazepines (Huang, Kutner, & Bliwise, 2009; Yeung, Chung, Zhang, Yap, & Law, 2009). However, these studies were deemed to have considerable issues related to bias and were of low quality. Therefore, acupuncture for insomnia is a somewhat promising treatment option, but no clear conclusion regarding efficacy or safety can be drawn as of yet. No randomized controlled trials have as yet examined the effects of massage on insomnia.

Mind–body interventions use techniques or approaches that are aimed at self-regulating the mind and body, typically to reduce stress-related symptoms. Many of the principles or techniques are based in Eastern traditions of healing, designed to promote a sense of calmness in the mind and body. These interventions are typically delivered in small groups led by a teacher who guides participants through activities. Yoga is one such activity that includes a series of postures and breathing regulation. Studies have shown that engagement in certain yoga practices can improve symptoms of insomnia, including increased TST, decreased total wake time in bed, and improvements in sleep quality (Khalsa, 2004). Tai chi is a form of Chinese martial arts involving a sequence of slow movements designed to enhance self-regulation of the mind and body. Tai chi appears to be particularly suitable for older adults, with evidence that tai chi was rated as superior by a health-education comparison group on self-reported sleep quality (Irwin, Olmstead, & Motivala, 2008). A comparative efficacy study found that tai chi was associated with improvements in sleep quality, fatigue, and depressive symptoms, but not remission of insomnia when compared with CBT-I (Irwin et al., 2014).

Perhaps the most promising mind–body intervention for insomnia is meditation. *Meditation* is a self-regulation practice that involves introspection and contemplation about a concept or mantra, usually to bring about a sense of calmness. Thus, meditation fits the conceptual model of reducing arousal related to insomnia. However, using a meditation practice to immediately induce sleep, similar to the mechanism of sleep medication, has not been shown to be effective for people with insomnia. Instead, it appears that the consistent practice of meditation can cultivate mental and physical states that can reduce the symptoms of a chronic insomnia disorder. Among the various types of meditation practices, mindfulness meditation has emerged as a recognized and viable meditation practice that is gaining popularity. The remainder of this book focuses on the use of mindfulness meditation for insomnia.

Mindfulness Meditation
Awakening to Better Sleep

3

This chapter provides an overview of mindfulness meditation and the principles of mindfulness that serve as the foundation for the mindfulness-based therapy for insomnia (MBTI) program. The goal is to provide MBTI instructors with a historical and philosophical background for understanding the mindfulness techniques that are described in Part II of this book. This chapter begins with definitions of terms related to the principles of mindfulness and the practice of mindfulness meditation, followed by an explanation of how mindfulness meditation can be applied as a means of self-regulation. The origins of mindfulness in Buddhist philosophy are discussed, and a historical context is provided with regard to mindfulness and third wave behavior therapies. Distinctions between the concept of mindfulness, meditation, and cognitive therapies are made to orient the reader to the similarities and differences between mindfulness-based therapies (MBTs), traditional cognitive behavior therapies (CBTs), and other types of third wave behavior therapies. A brief overview of the evidence of MBTs used for other

http://dx.doi.org/10.1037/14952-004
Mindfulness-Based Therapy for Insomnia, by J. C. Ong

health conditions (e.g., depression, eating disorders) is given to provide a broader context for how mindfulness meditation has been used to improve health in other areas.

What Is Mindfulness Meditation?

The concept of mindfulness is rooted in Buddhist philosophy, in which the term *mindfulness* means to "see with discernment" or to see the present moment clearly without judgment. Translations of the Buddhist term for mindfulness also encompass elements of awareness, circumspection, and self-compassion. It is important to note that the intention of being mindful is to cultivate awareness of the present moment that is not attached to a particular reason or outcome. Kabat-Zinn (1990) described *mindfulness* as paying attention in a specific way to distinguish this from situations in which paying attention is used to achieve a purpose or to analyze a situation. For the purposes of this book, *mindfulness* is broadly defined as an intentional act of present-moment awareness without attachment to outcomes.

There are several principles, or qualities, that are embodied during a state of mindfulness (Kabat-Zinn, 1990). These principles include non-judging, patience, nonstriving, letting go, acceptance, beginner's mind, and trust. *Nonjudging* refers to awareness without a preference; that is, without making judgments about thoughts as "good and bad" or "right and wrong." Being mindful is to be present with one's thoughts as they arise without attempting to focus on the "good" or avoid the "bad." *Patience* and *nonstriving* are important principles because mindfulness is an act that cannot be forced or hurried. Similarly, mindfulness embodies *letting go*, or allowing things to be as they are in nature. The principle of *acceptance* is often confused with giving up. In contrast, acceptance in this context is acknowledgment of what is present without the need to immediately fix the problem or make it better. *Beginner's mind* refers to approaching each moment with a clear perspective that is not clouded by past experiences. Finally, *trust* involves recognizing the importance of the self and having compassion for the self. These principles are the core of adopting a mindful approach to each moment. In Chapter 5, I discuss these principles in greater detail and explain how each can be applied to insomnia.

When people think of meditation, the most common image that comes to mind is that of an individual sitting with eyes closed, focusing his or her mind on a particular mental or physical activity. The activity might be a mantra, a prayer, clearing the mind, or focusing on breathing. This purpose of meditation might be of a religious nature or a process of transformation. Certainly, all of these could be considered forms of meditation, and indeed there are many different ways to meditate. In the context of mindfulness, meditation is seen as an activity that embodies attention, awareness, and compassion. As defined earlier, the attention and awareness are directed at the present moment. Compassion is cultivated by approaching the present moment with curiosity, kindness, and gentleness. This can be directed toward oneself as an act of self-compassion or toward others in the form of empathy and connection. As with most things, this takes practice. So *mindfulness meditation* can be defined as the practice of mindfulness awareness, compassion, and nonattachment to outcomes.

Although mindfulness can be practiced across different activities, it is important to note what mindfulness meditation does not entail. Mindfulness meditation is not simply another relaxation technique. Although one might well experience relaxation, it is not a direct goal of meditating in this context. Mindfulness meditation is also not about positive thinking. Recall that nonjudging is a key principle of mindfulness. Therefore, it is not about focusing on the positive experiences and avoiding the negative ones. It is important to be mindful of whatever is present, without trying to eliminate or avoid the negative experiences. Mindfulness is also not about trying to go into a trance or clearing the mind of all thoughts. The qualities of mindfulness are quite the opposite—they are about inviting all that is present to simply be present. In doing so, it is important not to resist or avoid any particular thought and not to transcend to a different mental state. There are other forms of meditation that have different philosophical principles. For example, transcendental meditation emphasizes the practice of concentrating attention on an object or word until the distinction between the subject (meditator) and object are one point in the mind. In contrast, mindfulness meditation emphasizes the insight gained from awareness of activities in the mind and body that occur from moment to moment. Rather than clearing the mind of all thoughts, it is about practicing how to work with thoughts that are present. These are some common misconceptions of MBTI that instructors should be familiar with and be able to discuss with participants.

WHY SHOULD ONE PRACTICE MINDFULNESS MEDITATION?

From the Buddhist tradition, the answer to this question is rooted in the basic Buddhist tenet that life is suffering and all beings suffer. Accordingly, the cause of the suffering is one's attachment to outcomes. In other words, the desire or craving to achieve a certain outcome is the root of our suffering. For example, we might be applying for a very desirable job. However, we are not in a position to control the outcome, so the desire to have the job creates stress, anxiety, and possibly depressed mood if we do not get it.

The practice of mindfulness meditation offers a way to relieve this suffering. By practicing mindfulness meditation, we draw our attention to the present-moment experience and allow ourselves to be patient, nonstriving, and accepting of outcomes (i.e., we get the job or we do not). All of these qualities allow us to let go of the attachment to the desired outcome. Long-term practice of mindfulness meditation allows us to become aware of the impermanence in nature—all things change. Awareness of this concept helps us understand that both internal and external states are dynamic and not fixed, and thus thoughts are not facts about the world but simply thoughts about our perception the world. Thus, the cause of the distress that was experienced by wanting the job of our choice, is itself a choice! We can choose to let go of our attachment or desire for a particular outcome, and this will relieve the distress that comes with that attachment. This process of awareness and reconceptualization of our thoughts and desires is what allows us to let go of our attachment to outcomes. By paying attention to the present moment and watching each moment pass, one can begin to see a situation or problem more clearly or become more "awakened" to a new solution. By embodying the principles of nonstriving, patience, acceptance, and trust, the practice of mindfulness meditation allows the mind to shift to a place where it does not have to suffer. This shift is seen as an act of self-compassion because we are allowing ourselves to release from the distress.

DOES MINDFULNESS MEDITATION TAKE SPECIALIZED TRAINING?

Earlier, I noted that the most common image of meditation is sitting quietly in a lotus position in a state of contemplation. Whereas this might be one form of mindfulness meditation practice, there are many ways to practice mindfulness. In addition to sitting meditations, it is possible to practice mindfulness meditation by lying down and mentally scanning different parts of the body to develop awareness of various thoughts and physical sensations. It is also possible to bring mindful awareness to movement through a walking meditation. Yoga and tai chi can also be forms of mindfulness meditation. Furthermore, it is possible to extend the practice of mindfulness to everyday living—riding a bike, working out, or even interacting with others. These can be considered informal meditations because they bring the principles of mindfulness to common activities of daily living as opposed to a designated time set aside for a formal meditation. Most important, mindfulness meditation does not have to be an esoteric activity reserved for Buddhist monks or for those who can afford to spend months in Tibet. The practice of mindfulness meditation can be done by anyone. However, most people will need help from an instructor to establish a formal meditation practice and to provide guidance on how to apply the principles of meditation to a particular situation or condition.

Indeed, meditation practice is the central "ingredient" in mindfulness-based programs. The practice of meditation provides an opportunity to cultivate the principles of mindfulness and such practice allows for a deeper sense of self-compassion and well-being. Therefore, it is important to develop and maintain a consistent meditation practice to cultivate the mindfulness principles. This applies to those participating in an MBTI program as well as MBTI instructors. Later, I discuss some of the issues related to MBTI instructors having a personal meditation practice.

The Rise of Mindfulness-Based Therapies in Western Cultures

Although mindfulness meditation has its origins in Eastern philosophy, it is now being taught in Western cultures through programs known as *mindfulness-based therapies* (MBTs). The original MBT was developed by Jon Kabat-Zinn, who is trained professionally as a microbiologist but also received personal training in Buddhist meditation. Kabat-Zinn (1990) developed a program known as *mindfulness-based stress reduction* (MBSR), an 8-week program that teaches participants how to begin and maintain a personal mindfulness meditation practice to help relieve stress and suffering related to medical conditions. The program was designed as a psychoeducation class and delivered in a group format. Over the years, Kabat-Zinn and colleagues have conducted several studies on MSBR that demonstrated the benefits of practicing mindfulness meditation. These benefits include improving psoriatic lesions (Kabat-Zinn et al., 1998), symptoms of anxiety (Koszycki, Benger, Shlik, & Bradwejn, 2007), high blood pressure (Hughes et al., 2013), and chronic pain (Schmidt et al., 2011). In particular, the benefits seemed to have sustainable long-term effects (Kabat-Zinn, Lipworth, Burney, & Sellers, 1987).

The success of MBSR led to the adaptation of MBTs for more specific health conditions. Mindfulness-based cognitive therapy (MBCT) was developed by Segal, Williams, and Teasdale (2002) as a program to prevent the relapse of depression among individuals with recurrent major depressive disorder. In their first randomized controlled trial, Segal and his colleagues found that MBCT was more effective than standard pharmacological treatment at reducing the risk of a relapse or recurrence of having a major depressive episode over a 60-week period for individuals with three or more previous episodes of depression. In a second study, Segal et al. (2010) found that MBCT was comparable to a pharmacological maintenance therapy in reducing relapse of depression over an 18-month period following remission after acute treatment for depression. Relative to a placebo pill, MBCT reduced the risk of relapse by 74%, whereas pharmacotherapy reduced the risk of relapse by 76%. Another MBT, *mindfulness-based eating awareness therapy*, is a program designed to help individuals with eating disorders and weight management (Kristeller & Hallett, 1999). There is also a mindfulness-based program for preventing relapse in alcohol and substance use (Witkiewitz, Marlatt, & Walker, 2005). Other forms of MBT have been used to reduce psychological symptoms and improve quality of life in several chronic diseases, including cancer (Carlson et al., 2013; Carlson & Speca, 2010), HIV/AIDS (Gonzalez-Garcia et al., 2013), fibromyalgia (Schmidt et al., 2011), heart disease (Hughes et al., 2013; Parswani, Sharma, & Iyengar, 2013), diabetes (van Son et al., 2013), and irritable bowel syndrome (Zernicke et al., 2013). All of these MBTs draw from the Buddhist lineage of mindfulness principles and teach meditation as a central component of the program. Recent data indicate that over 500 clinics worldwide now offer MBSR (Cullen, 2011), and a systematic review found 477 academic journal articles published on MBTs in 2013 (Black, 2014).

Given the large body of evidence now available for MBTs, several reviews and meta-analyses on treatment effectiveness have revealed a positive benefits-to-risk profile. Hofmann, Sawyer, Witt, and Oh (2010) found medium pre-to-post effect sizes on anxiety (Hedge's $g = 0.63$) and depression (Hedge's $g = 0.59$) overall, with larger effect sizes among clinical populations (Hedge's $g = 0.97$ for anxiety, 0.95 for depression). Khoury et al. (2013) examined effect sizes across different study designs and populations, revealing moderate effect sizes for MBTs in pre–post designs (Hedge's $g = 0.55$), MBTs compared with wait-list controls (Hedge's $g = 0.53$), and MBTs compared with psychoeducation controls (Hedge's $g = 0.61$). Smaller effects were found when MBTs were compared with supportive therapies ($g = 0.37$), imagery techniques ($g = 0.27$) and relaxation techniques ($g = 0.19$). No significant differences were found when MBTs were compared with behavior therapies ($g = -0.07$) or pharmacotherapy ($g = 0.13$). Finally, a recent meta-analysis on meditation programs supported by the Agency for Healthcare Research and Quality (Goyal et al., 2014) found that MBTs have moderate evidence for improving anxiety ($d = 0.38$) and depression ($d = 0.30$) at post-treatment and at 3- to 6-month follow-up ($d = 0.22$ for anxiety, $d = 0.23$ for depression). It is important to note that these effect sizes are comparable to effect sizes found for antidepressant medication ($d = 0.11–0.17$), but MBTs have fewer reported side effects (Goyal et al., 2014). Collectively, these data indicate that MBTs are viable programs for improving health.

Are Mindfulness-Based Therapies a Form of Psychotherapy or Alternative Medicine?

In reviewing the literature on the benefits of MBTs, most studies have focused on outcomes in mental health and well-being. As noted earlier, MBSR was originally developed as a psychoeducational class, not as a form of psychotherapy or a substitution for mental health care. During these early classes, Kabat-Zinn and his colleagues made this clear to participants. Those who had significant psychiatric conditions, such as posttraumatic stress disorder or bipolar depression, were allowed to participate only if they were stable, under the care of a mental health expert, or both. As other MBTs began to emerge, many of these adaptations were developed for specific populations, such as those with a history of depression or those with eating disorders. The movement toward clinical populations thus raises the question of whether or not MBTs are another form of psychotherapy or a form of alternative medicine.

At the conceptual level, mindfulness principles share many similarities with modern psychological theories, most notably with cognitive behavioral theories. The focus on mental activities as a cause of emotional distress is similar to cognitive theories of depression (Beck, Rush, Shaw, & Emery, 1979) and anxiety (Barlow, 2004). For example, rumination and negative thoughts about the self or the outside world are the core cognitive features of depression. In the case of anxiety, worries about the future or specific situations are difficult to control, leading to catastrophic thoughts or expectations. It is interesting to note that in both depression and anxiety, thoughts are often focused on the past or the future but not on the present.

Mindfulness principles bring similar attention to working with thoughts that can create a state of depression or anxiety. Rather than focusing on the content of the thoughts, the act of being mindful brings attention to one's relationship with the thoughts. Rather than judging the thoughts as good or bad, as rationale or irrational, the mindful approach is to simply acknowledge that the thoughts are present and to determine whether one might be able to decenter, reperceive, or relate differently to these thoughts rather than changing the thoughts themselves.

Another distinction between MBTs and psychotherapy involves the content of treatment. The techniques taught in both MBTs and CBTs are similar in that they first involve an assessment of the present situation and then use this assessment to reduce emotional distress (i.e., emotion-focused coping) or make behavioral changes (i.e., problem-focused coping). Within a CBT framework, emotion-focused coping involves techniques such as seeking social support, expressive writing, or emotional disclosure. These techniques can be similar or even considered mindful acts because they also involve changes at the cognitive level.

The contrast between MBT and CBT techniques begins with meditation. MBT is grounded in meditation, which serves as the core for practicing and embodying mindfulness principles. In CBT, there are often homework and specific tasks to practice that reinforce the lessons taught in session, but no specific focus on meditation. Second, both MBT and CBT involve techniques aimed at reducing emotional distress, but the method of achieving this differs. In MBT, the focus is on shifting the relationship with distressing thoughts. In some contexts, this has been considered to be targeting metacognitions, rather than cognitions. In contrast, traditional CBT, attempts to identify the maladaptive thought and to correct it through Socratic questioning. This involves challenging thoughts through a series of questions (e.g., Is this thought realistic? Is there evidence for it?), which usually involves making judgments of whether a thought is "rational" or "irrational." This approach is different from the nonjudgmental approach of being mindful of all thoughts. A second difference can be seen in specific techniques, such as the body scan (a quiet meditation) versus progressive muscle relaxation (PMR). In the body scan, the purpose is to cultivate awareness and stay present with whatever thoughts or body sensations arise in the moment as one is practicing this quiet meditation. In contrast, the purpose of PMR is to induce a relaxation response achieved through deep breathing and intentionally tightening and then relaxing the muscles. Thus, PMR has a particular goal, whereas the body scan meditation does not. A third difference can be seen in the overall approach to delivery of information. As a family of treatments, CBT tends to be didactic and outcome-oriented with various techniques used to track progress (e.g., events log) and evaluate outcomes with the goal of reducing specific symptoms or behaviors. In contrast, MBTs tend to be experiential and process-oriented, with the focus on the practice of meditation and discoveries or insights learned through meditation practice rather than monitoring symptom reduction. Table 3.1 summarizes the differences in techniques.

Another difference lies in the treatment providers. In traditional CBT, treatment is provided by a trained mental health expert, typically

TABLE 3.1

Comparison of Mindfulness-Based Therapies (MBTs) and Cognitive Behavior Therapies (CBTs)

Elements of treatment	MBT	CBT
Treatment targets	Shift relationship with thoughts and feelings (target = metacognitions)	Identify and challenge thoughts and/or behaviors that are maladaptive (target = cognitions/behaviors)
Intention of treatment activities	Cultivate awareness and stay present with whatever thoughts or body sensations arise in the moment (e.g., body scan)	Intent is to produce mental and physical relaxation (e.g., progressive muscle relaxation)
Treatment delivery	Experiential, process-oriented	Didactic, outcome-oriented

a psychologist, psychiatrist, clinical social worker, or psychiatric nurse. The level of training and expertise is often dictated by the clinical setting and nature of the patient's condition. In MBTs, treatment providers could be a psychologist, nurse, social worker, or physician, but one of the most essential prerequisites is that the provider has a personal meditation practice in order to fully embody mindfulness in teaching the MBT class. Also related to treatment providers is that CBT is typically covered under insurance plans that offer mental health coverage, whereas the status of MBTI is unclear. The issue of who is qualified to deliver MBTI and who should have access to MBTI is complex, and this controversy is discussed further in Chapter 10.

In conclusion, there are both similarities and differences between MBT and CBT in concepts, techniques, and providers of treatment. The point of these comparisons is not to make the case that one form of therapy is superior to the other but to clarify the unique elements of each. Some elements of MBT overlap with CBT, but I believe that MBT is distinct from CBT in certain conceptual approaches and treatment techniques. Some also see MBT as a progression in the lineage of behavior therapy, to CBT, and now rising as part of the third wave therapies, which include acceptance and commitment therapy, dialectical behavior therapy, and other metacognitive therapies. Although I have summarized the major points, the reader is directed to comments in the literature for further debates on this topic (Hayes, 2004; Hofmann, Sawyer, & Fang, 2010).

I would propose that MBT is a form of integrative medicine or integrative health intervention. *Integrative medicine* is defined as an approach to medicine that "reaffirms the importance of the relationship between practitioner and patient, focuses on the whole person, is informed by evidence, and makes use of all appropriate therapeutic approaches, health-care professionals and disciplines to achieve optimal health and healing" (Consortium of Academic Health Centers for Integrative Medicine, 2015). MBT fits this definition, as it avoids the distinction of "traditional medicine" versus "alternative medicine" and embodies a more inclusive definition that fits with the principles of mindfulness. Because most MBTs teach mindfulness meditation training along with some concepts that are usually derived from more modern theories from health psychology or medicine, the combination of these approaches would seem to fit the definition of integrative medicine. Notably, in January 2015, the National Institutes of Health changed the name for the National Center for Complementary and Alternative Medicine to the National Center for Complementary and Integrative Health, which has sponsored much of the research on mindfulness meditation and health.

PRINCIPLES AND PRACTICES OF MBTI

II

Theoretical Foundations and Preparation for MBTI

4

This chapter brings together the concepts described in Part I to explain the theory and concepts behind mindfulness-based therapy for insomnia (MBTI). The reader may wish to refer back to the relevant sections in the earlier chapters for review. This chapter prepares the instructor for delivering MBTI by discussing issues related to training, recruitment, and assessment of participants.

Theoretical Foundations of MBTI

PRINCIPLES AND PRACTICES FROM BEHAVIORAL SLEEP MEDICINE

Because MBTI was developed as a treatment for insomnia disorders, clinicians who wish to deliver MBTI should be familiar with several key theoretical models and concepts

http://dx.doi.org/10.1037/14952-005
Mindfulness-Based Therapy for Insomnia, by J. C. Ong

about sleep and insomnia. As mentioned in Chapter 1, these concepts relate to the distinction between acute sleep disturbance and chronic insomnia disorders that develop over several months. Recall that the triggers of acute sleep disturbance usually involve dysregulation in the systems that regulate sleep, stress, or both. The transformation of acute sleep disturbance into an insomnia disorder involves changes in sleep-related behaviors and cognitions that perpetuate the sleep disturbance and daytime dysfunction over the course of several weeks or months. The application of these concepts and models to mindfulness principles is reviewed in the following paragraphs.

Connecting the Two-Process Model of Sleep Regulation With Mindfulness Principles

The two-process model of sleep regulation (Borbély, 1982; Borbély & Achermann, 1999) was introduced in Chapter 1 and serves as the predominant model for understanding human sleep–wake regulation. This model of sleep regulation provides a foundation for understanding how the brain reacts to acute sleep disturbance caused by certain waking behaviors and then automatically regulates over time. An important connection between this model and MBTI is the concept that the brain is capable of regulating sleep on its own. Putting active effort or striving to make sleep happen is often counterproductive and can interfere with the systems in the brain. This concept is similar to breathing because the brain can regulate the depth and rate of breathing based on the situation. During normal activity, breathing is regular, with a consistent pace. When the situation requires a high level of activity, such as exercise, the rate of breathing increases and breaths become shorter. However, trying to exert conscious control over breathing can sometimes backfire, such as hyperventilating during an anxious situation. Although the two-process model has many intricacies that are beyond the scope of MBTI, it is important for an MBTI instructor to understand the basic concepts of Process S and Process C so that these can be explained in a way that patients can understand. Knowing that the brain is capable of regulating sleep on its own can also aid in reducing anxiety about sleep.

For explaining Process S to a patient, I often use the analogy to an appetite for food. I start by asking the patient the last time he or she ate a meal and use that as a guide for explaining how (under normal circumstances) with each amount of time that passes without food, the patient's appetite for food (i.e., hunger) will increase. In fact, going a period of time without food is the only behavioral way to increase the physical state of hunger. I then use this analogy to explain how we have an "appetite for sleep" (i.e., Process S), such that (under normal circumstances) going for a period of time without sleep is the only behavioral way to increase the physical state of sleepiness. One difference is that it takes a longer amount of time to generate a sufficient appetite for a full night of sleep compared with the amount of time needed to generate a sufficient appetite for food. The appetite for sleep builds across 16 to 18 hours of continuous wakefulness. In contrast, it usually takes only 4 to 6 hours to generate a sufficient appetite for eating a whole meal of food. Therefore, a key concept to convey to the patient is that Process S requires a sufficient amount of continuous wakefulness in order to generate a sufficient appetite for sleeping through the night. In other words, trying to sleep whenever possible and/or spending more time in bed are counterproductive behaviors that actually increase the likelihood of sleep disturbance. In MBTI, this behavior is seen as "avoiding wakefulness" because spending more time in bed becomes a means to escape or avoid being awake.

If Process S were the only mechanism that controlled sleep and wake, then the sleep period would only depend on the amount of wakefulness and it would not matter what time of day the sleep and wake periods occurred. However, humans sleep better at night, when it is dark, than during the day, when it is light. Recall that Process C regulates the timing of the sleep period, promoting sleep at night and activity during the day. There are two points of emphasis that are related to Process C. First, the rise time (i.e., time getting out of bed to start the day) is the key for setting the timing of the circadian rhythm. Most people think that the bedtime is the key, but the intrinsic timekeeper in the brain is most effective when the rise time is consistent across days with exposure to light shortly thereafter. Consequently, the common behavior of "sleeping in" to catch up on sleep (i.e., delaying the wake-up time when there is no need to wake up by a certain time) usually ends up being a counterproductive attempt to get more sleep because it disrupts Process C, making it more difficult to achieve regular sleep on future nights. The second point of emphasis is that melatonin is released about 1 to 2 hours before the regular bedtime, but this requires relatively dim light conditions. Recall from Chapter 1 that the release of melatonin signals the brain to turn off the wake-promoting systems and prepare for sleep. As a result, exposure to bright light can suppress melatonin release and cause the brain to continue in waking mode. Therefore, paying attention to the timing of our behaviors and establishing regular routines in the morning and evening can help Process C function optimally.

In summarizing how these two sleep–wake processes work, it is helpful to connect some of the mindfulness principles with sleep regulation. Even if sleep disruption occurs on any given night, MBTI instructors should encourage patients to trust in the brain's ability to self-regulate, have patience in allowing sleep to happen on its own, and avoid striving to fix the acute sleep disturbance. The essential message to communicate is that the brain is capable of regulating sleep if we do not interfere with it. It also reinforces the notion that resolving an insomnia disorder is a workable problem, but whether acute sleep disturbance will occur on any given night is not always controllable. This shifts the attention away from the attachment to seek solutions for immediate gains and to focus instead on regulation of sleep and daytime function across nights. Specific activities for delivering this message are discussed in the following chapters.

Connecting Models of Chronic Insomnia With Mindfulness Principles

Understanding the move from acute sleep disturbance to chronic insomnia brings with it the need to understand the development and maintenance of insomnia disorders. In Chapter 1, several influential models of chronic insomnia (Espie, 2002; Harvey, 2002; Morin, 1993; Perlis, Giles, Mendelson, Bootzin, & Wyatt, 1997; Spielman, Caruso, & Glovinsky, 1987) were reviewed, and MBTI instructors should be familiar with how these models conceptualize insomnia disorders. One theme that is consistent across these models is how *sleep effort* (i.e., the effort to make sleep better) plays a role in the development and maintenance of insomnia over time. In the 3-P model (Spielman et al., 1987), sleep effort involves perpetuating factors such as staying in bed or taking frequent naps. In Espie's (2002) psychobiological inhibition model, sleep effort involves selective attention to sleep and a failure to recognize appropriate cues to dearouse for sleep. In MBTI, sleep effort is seen as a distortion of the value of sleep within an individual's life. Whereas other treatments, such as cognitive behavior therapy for insomnia (CBT-I), address sleep effort through directly targeting cognitions or behaviors, MBTI addresses the problem indirectly by having participants observe and develop an awareness of the change in sleep effort and then allow the brain's sleep regulation system to restore sleep without forcing it to happen. Most conceptual models also emphasize the role of hyperarousal as a key etiological factor in maintaining the sleep disturbance over time (Espie, 2002; Morin, 1993; Perlis et al., 1997; Spielman et al., 1987). MBTI works with the problem by using awareness to address reactive tendencies of people with insomnia, such as the desire to quickly fix the sleep problem, that tend to exacerbate sleep-related arousal. Rather than changing the thought (e.g., challenging maladaptive cognitions) or the behavior (e.g., using progressive muscle relaxation) directly, MBTI is aimed at shifting the relationship with the thought or the behavior.

MBTI also builds on the models that conceptualize insomnia as a 24-hour problem, such that the treatment includes tools to address daytime dysfunction in addition to sleep-specific symptoms. One central theme in MBTI is the conceptualization of insomnia as not only a sleep problem but also a condition that encompasses many other domains. The *territory of insomnia* is a term used to highlight the range of domains that insomnia can encompass. In addition to the nocturnal symptoms, such as difficulty falling and staying asleep, the territory of insomnia includes the impact of insomnia on daytime behaviors, thoughts and attitudes about sleep, and metacognitions related to sleep (which are discussed later in this chapter). In other words, it goes beyond the clinical criteria for insomnia and includes behavioral, cognitive, and metacognitive aspects that can arise during the course of chronic insomnia. In Chapter 7, I explain how unveiling this wider "territory" can provide a more comprehensive map to identify particular areas that might require attention.

PRINCIPLES AND PRACTICES FROM MINDFULNESS MEDITATION AND THIRD WAVE BEHAVIOR THERAPIES

Concepts From Buddhist Philosophy

As a mindfulness-based therapy, MBTI is grounded in the principles of Buddhist philosophy and mindfulness meditation, which were presented in Chapter 3, and applies these concepts to work with the problem of insomnia. Recall that mindfulness is a state of intentionally bringing one's awareness to the present moment in a nonjudgmental manner (Kabat-Zinn, 1990) and that this state involves the embodiment of seven principles: beginner's mind, nonstriving, letting go, nonjudging, acceptance, trust, and patience. I discussed earlier how the principles of trust, patience, and nonstriving can be used to explain why most efforts to improve sleep are counterproductive and actually perpetuate the problem. The principle of beginner's mind is important for avoiding the trap that the previous night's poor sleep will necessarily have a negative impact on the present night's sleep when, in fact, it will probably have a positive impact on tonight's sleep. The principles of letting go, nonjudging, and acceptance are important for reducing sleep-related arousal by cultivating awareness of the problem in a nonbiased manner and minimizing the tendency to be reactive problem solvers. Mindfulness is also associated with the self-compassion that is cultivated when an individual practices mindfulness skills across numerous situations in daily living. The practice of mindfulness meditation involves observing the mind's contents with discernment. This involves training in the placement of attention while being fully present in each moment. Therefore, mindfulness is an inherent ability that lies within all human beings, but practice is required to access this ability. MBTI is designed to help individuals who are willing to learn and practice these principles and skills.

Recall that impermanence is a central theme in Buddhism, such that all material things come and go, and the attachment to a desired outcome is the root cause of emotional distress. In the context of MBTI, sleeplessness is viewed as a transient state and the attachment to sleeping better becomes the root cause of sleep-related distress in an insomnia disorder. This attachment leads to rigidity and a restricted range in one's responses to sleep disturbance. In MBTI, mindful meditation practice is designed to enhance the ability to respond to mental and physical states associated with insomnia using a wider range of options, rather than reacting to them in the rigid, ineffective manner that has perpetuated the insomnia disorder. Like other mindfulness-based therapies, MBTI is based on the idea that cultivating intentional awareness of the present moment, self-compassion, and nonattachment to outcomes can aid in alleviating mental and physical distress by accepting the present state and responding with intention and mindfulness rather than reacting automatically with mindlessness (Kabat-Zinn, 1990). Rather than changing the environment or source of stress, mindfulness meditation promotes changing the individual's relationship with stress. In this way, there is a shift from an outcome-oriented approach (actions to relieve stress) to a process-oriented approach (observing that stress is present) that focuses on metacognitions.

Integration of Mindfulness Principles With Modern Psychology

Modern psychology has adopted many principles of mindfulness from Buddhism and reconceptualized them within existing frameworks that involve stress and the process of psychopathology. Teasdale (1999), well-known for his work in mood disorders, explained how facilitating metacognitive insight can be used to prevent the relapse of depression. By teaching the idea that thoughts are not facts but events in the mind, he demonstrated that practicing mindfulness could achieve metacognitive insight to those prone to experiencing recurring depressive episodes. He and his colleagues introduced the term *decentering*, which is defined as the ability to "step outside" of one's immediate experience, thereby changing the very nature of that experience (Segal, Williams, & Teasdale, 2002). Decentering involves a metacognitive shift in that the change is with the experience, not the thought itself. This important feature is one aspect that distinguishes Teasdale's approach from other forms of cognitive therapy, such as Beck's approach (Beck, Rush, Shaw, & Emery, 1979).

A similar model applied more broadly was proposed by Shapiro and colleagues, who called their model the *IAA model*, in which intention, attention, and attitude (IAA) are seen as interwoven processes that can lead to "reperceiving" experiences (Shapiro, Carlson, Astin, & Freedman, 2006). Another model examining the role of metacognitions in stress appraisal and coping was proposed by Garland, Gaylord, and Park (2009). Applying the concept of metacognitions to the Lazarus and Folkman (1984) stress and coping model, Garland et al. (2009) proposed that a mode of mindfulness allows one to decenter from the primary, or initial, stress appraisal and that this facilitates reappraisal with a different perspective that can promote more positive attributes. This new mindful reappraisal is hypothesized to attenuate the stress reaction (e.g., activation of the hypothalamic–pituitary–adrenal axis) and to cultivate positive emotions rather than to suppress negative emotions. Therefore, mindfulness might potentiate the capacity for positive reappraisal as an active coping strategy.

These models demonstrate how mindfulness principles can be integrated into modern psychological theories on cognitions and behaviors. Specifically, these models focus on the shift in mental processes rather than a direct change in the mental contents or behaviors. This shift in perspective (stance) enhances self-regulation and promotes an adaptive response (action), rather than maladaptive stress reactivity (reaction). Because these do not target the thoughts themselves, but rather the way one relates to these thoughts, they take on a broad, contextual approach to changing mental functioning.

METACOGNITIVE MODEL OF INSOMNIA

My colleagues Rachel Manber and Christi Ulmer and I have developed a conceptual model of insomnia that builds on the concepts from behavioral sleep medicine (BSM) and mindfulness meditation that we call the *metacognitive model of insomnia* (Ong, Ulmer, & Manber, 2012). In this model, we propose adding a layer of metacognition to the existing cognitive, behavioral, and physiological layers of insomnia that previous models have proposed (see Figure 4.1). We distinguish *metacognitions* from *cognitions* in that the former use two levels of sleep-related cognitive arousal and the latter use one—primary arousal. *Primary arousal* consists of the cognitive activity directly related to the inability to sleep. This includes the thoughts that interfere with sleep and the beliefs about daytime consequences of poor or insufficient sleep. Primary arousal includes maladaptive beliefs and attitudes about sleep (Morin, Stone, Trinkle, Mercer, & Remsberg, 1993) and sleep-interfering thoughts (Lundh & Broman, 2000). In addition to primary arousal, we propose another level, *secondary arousal*, which consists of how one relates to sleep-related thoughts. This includes the emotional valence one assigns to those thoughts, the degree of attachment one has to them, and the meaning or interpretation of

FIGURE 4.1

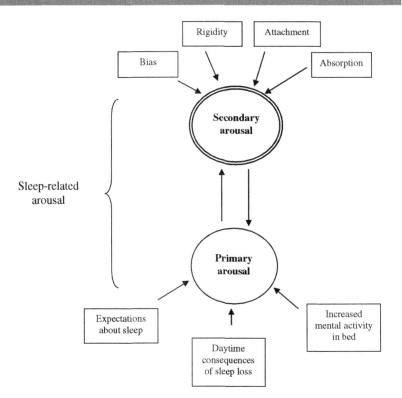

Metacognitive model of insomnia. From "Improving Sleep With Mindfulness and Acceptance: A Metacognitive Model of Insomnia," by J. C. Ong, C. S. Ulmer, and R. Manber, 2012, *Behaviour Research and Therapy*, 50, p. 653. Copyright 2012 by Elsevier. Adapted with permission.

those thoughts in relation to one's values. Therefore, secondary arousal involves negative metacognitions that often arise from the attachment and desire to satisfy sleep needs and tends to amplify the negative emotional valence or create a bias in the attention to and perception of sleep-related thoughts at the primary level. For example, the thought "I need 8 hours of sleep to function well the next day" can create primary arousal when the individual is lying in bed unable to sleep. A rigid attachment to this thought and a refusal to consider or accept alternative beliefs can amplify the valence, or degree of negative affect, associated with the thought, thereby creating secondary arousal. The degree to which one accepts thoughts as facts determines the valence these thoughts generate. Without the flexibility to allow competing thoughts to be considered (e.g., "I can find other ways to cope if I get less than 8 hours"), secondary arousal becomes a mechanism by which insomnia is perpetuated. The metacognitive model posits that both primary and secondary arousal should be seen as factors that promote and maintain the insomnia disorder across the daytime and nighttime.

Metacognitive processes are implicit in other models of insomnia, including the loss of automaticity described by Espie (2002), the selective attention given to sleep described by Harvey (2002), and the interpretive value of negative beliefs and attitudes about sleep discussed in Morin's (1993) model. Our metacognitive model is similar to the sleep-interpreting process, reflecting an interpretation of the immediate experience of thoughts and feelings about insomnia, proposed by Lundh and Broman (2000). However, these earlier models do not conceptualize metacognitive processes as distinct from other cognitive processes. We believe that the construct of metacognitions and secondary arousal provides greater specificity that can inform the maintenance of chronic insomnia. Furthermore, the concept of metacognitions can also be used to identify targets of treatment.

APPLICATION OF THE METACOGNITIVE MODEL IN MBTI

The MBTI treatment model uses the metacognitive model of insomnia to conceptualize sleep-related cognitive hyperarousal and failure to deactivate as central processes in the development and maintenance of insomnia. Using the concepts of primary and secondary arousal, the experience of insomnia is reconceptualized in the MBTI program as consisting of two levels of distress. *First-order distress* is about the actual impact of sleep loss, such as impairments in cognitive functioning or increased sleepiness. *Second-order distress* arises from the attachment and desire to satisfy sleep needs and tends to alter perception of sleep-related stress and amplify the first-order distress. Both first- and second-order distress are factors that promote and maintain the insomnia disorder. In MBTI, metacognitions are the primary targets for treatment by reducing sleep-related distress through second-order change.

The process of second-order change can be considered a metacognitive transformation or shift. Specifically, mindfulness meditation has the aim of increasing awareness of the mental and physical states that arise when experiencing insomnia symptoms and learning how to shift mental processes to promote an adaptive stance to one's responses to these symptoms. This stance is characterized by balanced appraisals of sleep expectations and the causes of daytime dysfunction, increased cognitive flexibility in approaching the symptoms of insomnia, nonattachment to sleep-related outcomes, and recommitting to values that are important to the individual. This new stance is posited to reduce arousal and prevent the perpetuation of negative emotions and behaviors that fuel the cycle of chronic insomnia. The process of metacognitive transformation is described in the following paragraphs.

Metacognitive Awareness

During an episode of insomnia, the strong attachment to sleep and the accompanying deficits that come with sleep deprivation can create an intense feeling of desperation. Patients are typically unaware of their own maladaptive cognitive, emotional, and behavioral reactions to sleep disturbance. I often hear patients saying, "All I want to do is sleep!" Such a response reflects a very mindless state with a desperate attachment to the outcome of sleeping that results in past-oriented thinking (e.g., "What could I have done to make my sleep better?") or future-oriented thinking (e.g., "How can I function tomorrow if I don't get any sleep tonight?"). There is a strong focus on the potential short-term negative consequences of poor sleep with responses directed at avoiding such consequences. The negative emotions created by the strong attachment to sleeping can bias the interpretation of the situation. Several studies have found that people with insomnia tend to be poor estimators of the amount of time they are sleeping in bed (Manconi et al., 2010; Tang & Harvey, 2005), and this deficit does not appear to be the result of a diminished ability to estimate time in general (Fichten, Creti, Amsel, Bailes, & Libman, 2005; Tang & Harvey, 2005). Earlier classification systems even included a subtype of insomnia that was called *sleep-state misperception* and later called *paradoxical insomnia* to describe the subgroup of insomnia patients whose main feature is a marked discrepancy between the subjective perception of sleep (e.g., self-reported data) and the objective measurement of sleep (e.g., through an overnight evaluation in a sleep lab). Most important, many patients will say things such as, "I seem to have forgotten how to fall asleep," meaning that they are no longer able to recognize the body's signals of sleepiness. Instead, they decide when to go to bed based on rules (e.g., "I should go to bed before midnight") or retire to bed to reduce mental and physical fatigue. Altogether, the poor awareness of their mental and physical state leads to increased effort to sleep, reactivity to sleep disturbance, and attachment to satisfying immediate sleep needs.

One of the first goals in MBTI is to establish a personal meditation practice. The reason for doing so is to cultivate mindfulness principles to develop greater awareness of the scope of the insomnia problem. By expanding awareness to include metacognitions, a patient with insomnia can begin to see how secondary arousal has contributed to their insomnia problem and how the attachment to sleeping better has created second-order distress. The cultivation of mindfulness promotes metacognitive awareness by allowing one to see the problem of insomnia with a clear lens that is not clouded by the desire and effort to sleep. Patients will sometimes comment on how they did not realize how reactive they had been and how these reactions had become so automatic, or mindless. Thus, metacognitive awareness provides a means to "awaken" the individual to his or her sleep-related experiences and facilitate insight into the problem rather than perpetuating the problem with mindless automatic reactions. The ability to cultivate metacognitive awareness then serves as the platform for taking intentional, mindful action as opposed to continuing in a state of automatic reactivity.

Metacognitive Shifting

After individuals develop metacognitive awareness, the practice of mindfulness principles challenges them to step outside of their own view of the problem and gain distance by taking an objective perspective. By shifting to an objective perspective that is outside of the desire to sleep, one is able to separate the experience of not sleeping (primary arousal) from the emotional attachment of seeking sleep (secondary arousal). *Metacognitive shifting* involves changing the relationship with thoughts rather than the content of thoughts. Instead of judging how realistic a thought might be and whether it is worth keeping, achieving mindful awareness promotes a metacognitive shift toward a more objective, nonjudging stance toward the thoughts themselves. This provides a platform from which to observe mental events as they are rather than trying to fix them.

In MBTI, metacognitive shifting consists of dearousal at the secondary level, which involves a shift in the relationship with sleep-related thoughts (i.e., the assigned degree of importance and the meaning or value of sleep) rather than directly changing the behaviors or thoughts associated with it, as is typically done in CBT-I. This shift can provide insight into patterns of mental and physical states that arise during the course of insomnia. For example, it could lead to the insight that the absorption in the frustration of not sleeping when desired (secondary arousal), rather than not sleeping itself (primary arousal), is the source of sleep-related distress. This shift follows the insight gained from metacognitive awareness and allows one to have greater equanimity, or a balanced emotional perspective, about the problem rather than trying to immediately change what is not desired.

New Metacognitive Stance

Metacognitive awareness and shifting leads to adoption of a new metacognitive stance. This new stance is characterized by balance, flexibility, equanimity, and a commitment to values that occur when the principles of mindfulness are embodied. Such a stance is an adaptive process

TABLE 4.1

Metacognitive Treatment Model for Insomnia

Elements of secondary arousal	Shift to adaptive stance	Reduction in secondary arousal
Attention and emotional bias toward sleep-seeking or sleep-aversive thoughts and behaviors	Balance	Allow the state of sleepiness to guide sleep-related behavior
Rigidity in sleep-related behaviors and beliefs	Flexibility	Adjusting intentionally to changing conditions
Attachment to sleep-related needs and expectations	Equanimity	Calmness stemming from non-striving and patience about sleep
Absorption in solving the sleep problem	Commitment to Values	Pursuit of valued living in the context of the range of thoughts and emotions

Note. From "Improving Sleep With Mindfulness and Acceptance: A Metacognitive Model of Insomnia," by J. C. Ong, C. S. Ulmer, and R. Manber, 2012, *Behaviour Research and Therapy, 50*, p. 655. Copyright 2012 by Elsevier. Adapted with permission.

that takes considerable work. It is typically an iterative process, involving frequent interactions among awareness, shifting, and adopting new stances. The key elements of an adaptive stance are summarized in Table 4.1 and described in more detail in the following paragraphs.

Balance

A balanced metacognitive stance involves managing the attraction and aversion to sleep. Many individuals with insomnia are "sleep seekers," meaning they have an imbalance in thoughts and behaviors of wanting sleep, such as striving to go to sleep or "clinging" to the bed in hopes of getting more sleep. Having balance with respect to sleep-related thoughts and behaviors can allow one to focus on the physical cues related to sleepiness as a guide for when to go to bed and when to wake up. This can enhance self-efficacy by aligning sleep-related behaviors with internal cues of sleepiness.

Flexibility

People with insomnia tend to demonstrate rigidity in their beliefs about sleep and their behavioral routines associated with sleeping. For example, people with insomnia have firm beliefs about the amount of sleep they need and the consequences that will occur when they do not receive adequate sleep (Morin et al., 1993). For them, there exists a cause-and-effect relationship that precludes any alternative outcomes. Behaviorally, people with insomnia often adopt specific routines or rituals that must be done to fall asleep. Harvey (2002) described these as *safety behaviors*, in the same way that people who suffer obsessive–compulsive disorder engage in safety behaviors as a means of coping with discomfort. An example of a safety behavior for some patients with insomnia is avoiding social functions at night because of the belief that staying out late causes insomnia. These rigid thoughts and behaviors reflect an unwillingness to accept sleeplessness and its consequences.

In contrast, a flexible metacognitive stance is characterized by qualities related to openness to what is happening in the present moment, willingness to adopt a beginner's mind, and acceptance of a wide range of cognitive and emotional phenomena. Approaching both the nighttime and daytime with a beginner's mind requires letting go of the contingencies that are based on expectations (e.g., the previous night's sleep or worries about the following day) and allowing the present night (or day) to unfold. Flexibility increases one's ability to let go of the rigid routines or thoughts that are fused with consequences and decreases secondary arousal.

Equanimity

Equanimity refers to a metacognitive stance that embodies composure and emotional centeredness with respect to sleep and sleep-related stimuli. This quality reflects a sense of calmness even when sleep is not happening as desired. In contrast, people with insomnia tend to have a strong emotional bias in the appraisal and perception of sleep-related stimuli. In one of our research studies, we found that poor sleepers, compared with good sleepers, report more negative emotional valence both in the daytime and the nighttime and more arousal at nighttime but not daytime (Ong, Cardé, Gross, & Manber, 2011). People with insomnia are also more likely to appraise stressful events as negative, despite a lack of significant differences in the frequency of stressful events (Friedman, Brooks, Bliwise, Yesavage, & Wicks, 1995; Morin, Rodrigue, & Ivers, 2003).

With equanimity, one adopts a stance that is nonstriving, composed, and patient and that facilitates improved emotion regulation in the face of insufficient sleep and fatigue. This stance can help to reduce the emotional bias that develops during the course of insomnia, by actively letting go of the desire to get a certain amount of sleep and letting go of the strong belief in contingencies between sleep and daytime functioning. It is important to note that this shift is an active strategy and does not involve suppression of thoughts. Nonattachment from this perspective does not imply a lack of feelings or emotions, but rather it suggests creating a space between a stimulus and the reaction to the stimulus. For example, letting go of the need to sleep 8 hours per night does not mean that one should no longer have thoughts about sleep needs. Rather, these thoughts shift toward how one feels at the present moment, and the recognition that thoughts about sleep are just thoughts about sleep, and nothing more, allowing the secondary arousal to dissipate. The shift toward equanimity is from the outcome (sleep) to the process (mental and physical sensations in the present moment), which serves to regulate the process of falling asleep.

Commitment to Values

Individuals experiencing chronic insomnia may lose sight of their values in life as their focus becomes more directed toward control of sleeplessness. With increasing anxiety about sleep, concessions are made to their values in the service of symptom management. For example, an individual who values health may forgo the morning exercise routine to compensate for a poor night of sleep by sleeping in late the next morning. In MBTI, increased awareness of nonsleep values can enhance willingness to enact behavioral recommendations for improving sleep, such as getting out of bed at the same time every day and letting go of ineffective and maladaptive strategies for dealing with insomnia (e.g., rigid thoughts and behaviors). Awareness of values can be a reference point for developing value-congruent goals and for determining whether individual actions are consistent with values. As such, MBTI adopts a value-based approach that encourages people to commit to actions that are value-congruent, even following a poor night of sleep. In this way, they can see the "big picture" (i.e., making value-congruent decisions in their lives) despite the perception of "losing battles" (i.e., getting less than ideal sleep) on any particular night.

Preparation for MBTI

Delivering MBTI requires certain levels of preparation and training for clinicians to be most effective. Whereas the beginning of this chapter focused on the conceptual aspects of MBTI, this section discusses the practical aspects of preparing to be an MBTI instructor and delivering MBTI.

PERSONAL TRAINING FOR DELIVERING MBTI

Because MBTI is a new program, there are currently no specific guidelines for the training to teach it. However, there are two qualifications that I feel are most important for clinicians who wish to deliver MBTI. First, it is essential that MBTI instructors have a personal meditation practice. This is a prerequisite for instructors who teach mindfulness-based stress reduction (MBSR), mindfulness-based cognitive therapy (MBCT), and most other mindfulness-based therapies, and I believe that MBTI should follow suit. The reason for this requirement is that the principles of mindfulness are best learned through one's own meditation practice. When instructors have a personal practice, they are more genuine in embodying these principles in their everyday lives and while teaching MBTI. Mindfulness principles are not a switch that can be turned on during MBTI and then turned off after the session has ended. Having a personal meditation practice helps instructors to keep mindfulness principles alive in all aspects of their lives, not just while teaching. Instructors who embody mindfulness demonstrate the qualities of living with mindfulness principles and taking value-congruent actions that can help participants connect with these principles and practices. Readers who are new to mindfulness meditation might consider engaging in training opportunities such as meditation retreats or professional workshops on meditation. These are discussed further in Chapter 10.

Earlier, I described how my personal experiences led to the realization of the importance of maintaining a personal practice. Segal, Williams, and Teasdale (2002) experienced a similar revelation when they were developing MBCT. They described how they initially believed that mindfulness might best fit into cognitive therapy. However, after two visits to observe MBSR classes taught by Kabat-Zinn and Santorelli, they found that teaching mindfulness was quite different from the "therapy mode" of collaboratively fixing problems with patients that is typically found in cognitive behavior therapy. Instead of fixing problems, MBSR instructors invited patients to take a more "allowing" or "welcoming" stance toward their problems and to observe what happened. The ways that MBSR instructors handled these issues were consistent with the practice of meditation, and thus the interactions between instructors and patients became another opportunity to embody and practice mindfulness principles. Hence, Segal, Williams, and Teasdale's conception of mindfulness was quite different in their final MBCT program.

The second qualification for teaching MBTI is to have some background or training in BSM. No specific board certification, program, or course is required. The information in this book can serve as a starting point, and additional courses, workshops, and/or continuing education activities in BSM can also be very useful (See Chapter 10 for resources). The rationale for this qualification is that a solid understanding of sleep physiology, and of behaviors and conditions that are productive and counterproductive for sleep, can help to cultivate patience and trust that sleep will happen and that the brain is capable of regulating sleep if we allow it to do so. This is important for the MBTI instructor to understand so that he or she can effectively communicate the process to patients.

Because MBTI is specifically designed to help people with insomnia, instructors should have appropriate credentials for working with a clinical population. Ideally, this would include a degree from a master's or doctoral-level training program and a professional license to deliver mental health or medical care. Some mindfulness-based programs, such as MBSR, are less restrictive and allow unlicensed providers to serve as instructors. As is discussed in Chapter 3, MBSR is positioned as a general psychoeducational program, whereas MBTI is a specialized program designed for a clinical condition. Therefore, psychologists who deliver MBTI should follow the American Psychological Association's (2010) *Ethical Principles of Psychologists and Code of Conduct*, which establishes standards for clinical practice. Other professionals should follow their own professional code of ethics for competency in delivering clinical services. Competency is discussed further in Chapter 10.

MATERIALS AND RESOURCES TO PREPARE FOR MBTI

In addition to the training background, MBTI instructors should take time to make sure that the materials and resources they need are in place and ready. The basic supplies that are needed include the following:

- Yoga mats: Providing yoga mats for participants helps to reduce the burden for them to bring their own mats to the MBTI sessions. Note that some participants might already own a mat and prefer to bring their own.
- Meditation chime, bell, or bowl: This is used by the instructor to signify the end of the meditation.
- Calculators: Calculators are used in Sessions 4 through 8 to compute sleep efficiency as part of the sleep consolidation program.
- Handouts: Having handouts helps reinforce mindfulness principles and homework practices. These should be prepared ahead of each session. Sample handouts and materials for each of the sessions are provided in the Appendix.
- Resource for home meditation practice: To help participants establish and maintain a home meditation practice, it is important to provide a resource such as digital media (i.e., CD, downloadable files) with guided meditations. Some instructors choose to create their own guided meditations, whereas others use established resources, such as the guided meditations by Kabat-Zinn.
- Food or water: This is optional, depending on the time that the MBTI group meets. In general, having groups in the evening tends to accommodate more participants. If the MBTI group is held around dinnertime, when participants are likely to be hungry, having light snacks might be helpful. A planned snack time can also provide an opportunity to practice mindful eating.

In addition to these materials, a large room is needed to conduct MBTI. The size of the room depends on the number of participants in the class. Ideally, the space can be configured as needed, with furniture that can be rearranged to allow sufficient room for participants to spread out during yoga and walking meditation. Large classrooms with folding chairs work well, whereas conference rooms with large tables tend to be less accommodating.

CONSIDERATIONS FOR SELECTING AND RECRUITING PATIENTS

Conducting Pre-MBTI Assessments

Given the variety of contexts in which MBTI might be delivered, some patients might be referred to MBTI after receiving a comprehensive sleep assessment, whereas other patients will have had no previous screening for sleep disorders or other medical and psychiatric conditions. Furthermore, some MBTI providers, such as those who work in sleep disorders or mental health clinics, will be able to independently conduct an assessment for insomnia as part of their practice. Other MBTI providers might receive referrals from a specialty clinic, thus relying on the referral source to conduct the assessment for insomnia. Although a comprehensive assessment of insomnia and other sleep disorders is beyond the scope of this book, MBTI instructors should conduct a basic prescreening assessment for all participants to determine suitability for participating in MBTI. As a guideline, the pre-MBTI assessment should address the following two clinical domains.

First, an assessment of the patient's sleep patterns and daytime functioning should be conducted to determine whether she or he meets criteria for an insomnia disorder. Questions should be aimed at characterizing the nocturnal insomnia symptoms, the daytime consequences of the nocturnal symptoms, and the history of the sleep pattern (e.g., number of insomnia episodes, frequency of symptom patterns). The reader is referred to Chapter 1 to review the diagnostic criteria for insomnia. As a reminder, MBTI is designed for people who are experiencing chronic insomnia and particularly for people who show symptoms of conditioned arousal associated with the sleep disturbance. Therefore, those who experience only occasional sleep disturbance, or those who meet criteria for acute insomnia, might be better suited for other treatment options, such as a brief behavior therapy for insomnia or sleep medication.

Second, assessment should be conducted to examine any urgent or severe comorbid conditions that should be addressed prior to initiating MBTI or that may require a different treatment altogether. In addition to assessing for insomnia symptoms, the assessment should include questions about other psychiatric and medical conditions. A brief review using a symptom checklist that contains key symptoms of a comorbid condition can be an efficient assessment tool. As noted earlier, the most common psychiatric comorbidities include mood and anxiety disorders. If comorbid mood disorders are present, assessment should focus on the severity and intensity of the symptoms to gauge whether the patient is capable of engaging in MBTI at this time or whether the mood disorder should be treated beforehand. Similarly, if other comorbid conditions are present, the MBTI instructor should assess the severity of the symptoms and their potential impact on the patient's ability to engage in MBTI. Notably, other sleep disorders, such as obstructive sleep apnea and circadian rhythm sleep disorders, also include insomnia symptoms as a presenting complaint. The presence of sleep apnea is usually indicated by symptoms such as snoring, witnessed pauses in breathing, and morning dry mouth and is accompanied by risk factors such as an elevated body mass index. If patients report these symptoms, then a referral to a sleep disorders clinic might be needed to rule out sleep apnea. Evaluation of longitudinal sleep patterns using 1 to 2 weeks of sleep diaries can determine sleep–wake patterns that are suggestive of an advanced or delayed sleep phase disorder.

In most cases, the pre-MBTI assessment requires only a clinical interview. Additionally, sleep diaries and other questionnaires that assess for comorbid medical and psychiatric conditions can be used to supplement the clinical interview. For example, having patients complete 1 or 2 weeks of sleep diaries prior to the pre-MBTI screening can help determine whether the sleep patterns meet criteria for chronic insomnia. Also, a checklist of symptoms can be completed by the patient and then used as part of the assessment for comorbid conditions. The importance of using additional tools is dictated by the setting and nature of the population.

As reported later in Chapter 9, our research thus far has been conducted only on people who do not have other sleep disorders or other uncontrolled psychiatric or medical conditions. We also have not tested MBTI on people who are taking sleep medications. That is not to say that these individuals are not appropriate candidates for MBTI, but rather that we do not yet have evidence about the benefits and risks of delivering MBTI for individuals with these considerations. Without an empirical basis for determining who is an appropriate candidate for MBTI, instructors are encouraged to use their own judgment with regard to skill level, experience, and expertise. For example, a licensed clinical psychologist or clinical social worker might be positioned to work with individuals who have insomnia and comorbid psychiatric conditions. Nurses or physicians might be capable of working with those who have comorbid medical conditions or those who are on sleep medications. Readers who wish to learn more about conducting assessments on insomnia should consult other resources that provide more detailed guidance on conducting comprehensive assessments (Buysse, Ancoli-Israel, Edinger, Lichstein, & Morin, 2006; Wyatt, Cvengros, & Ong, 2012).

MBTI Group Size

Instructors should also be cognizant of managing the group size for MBTI. In general, group sizes that range from six to eight individuals are optimal in terms of interpersonal considerations, management of group dynamics, and logistics of space and time management. When groups are smaller than four participants, the dynamics of the group can be greatly impacted if two or three people are absent or do not complete the program. Groups that are larger than 10 individuals can make it difficult to manage time and could result in some individuals feeling that their problems are not adequately addressed. These guidelines are similar to those used in other forms of group therapy. In determining the appropriate group size, instructors are again urged to use their own judgments of their group management skills, capabilities, and resources.

Getting Started With MBTI

5

A t the beginning of mindfulness-based therapy for insomnia (MBTI), most participants describe meditation as a quiet activity during which the eyes are closed and attention is brought to a single idea or to try and clear the mind of thinking. Some would also describe this as a way to cultivate positive affect, such as happiness or tranquility. In addition, many people would say that this is a special activity requiring a separate time set aside to practice, much like a prayer or religious ritual. Although all of these characterizations could describe meditation, mindfulness meditation has a particular intent and purpose in MBTI.

MBTI begins with an introduction to the concept of mindfulness through experiential activities to demonstrate that mindfulness meditation is not a special activity but a way of living. The program moves quickly into brief informal meditations to demonstrate how it is possible to be mindful with common activities, such as eating or breathing. Metaphors are used to illustrate the conceptual themes and connect them with real-life activities. In addition, it is emphasized that this

http://dx.doi.org/10.1037/14952-006
Mindfulness-Based Therapy for Insomnia, by J. C. Ong

approach is not a way to "meditate oneself to sleep." In other words, many people begin the program thinking that they will learn how to clear the mind, relax, and peacefully drift to sleep. In fact, they are quite surprised to learn that mindfulness meditation is a simple concept but one that requires considerable work. They are even more surprised to learn that meditation will not put them to sleep, but rather that they will be "awakened" from the mindless mode that is more typical in their current lives. At the end of the MBTI program, most people remark, "This isn't what I thought I would be doing."

This chapter describes the first two sessions of MBTI. The goals of the first two sessions are to (a) introduce the principles of MBTI, including the purpose of mindfulness meditation and the concepts that distinguish chronic insomnia from acute sleep disturbances; (b) provide instructions for establishing a meditation practice; and (c) develop awareness of the mental and physical states that arise during the course of insomnia. The meditation exercises, metaphors, discussions about insomnia, and daily monitoring of sleep and wakefulness activities serve as the modality for cultivating this awareness. In particular, mindful attention is brought to the mental and physical states that arise during the course of chronic insomnia, including sleepiness, fatigue, and hyperarousal. Participants are taught to mindfully observe these states without trying to immediately fix them. The establishment of a meditation practice is the key to developing a greater awareness of sleep-related behaviors (e.g., bedtime, wake time, activities in bed) and sleep-related thoughts (e.g., worries about not getting sufficient sleep). Awareness of these behaviors and thoughts is used to make new choices in sleep-related behaviors (described in Chapter 6) and sleep-related metacognitions (described in Chapter 7) later in the MBTI program. A general overview of the themes and key activities by each session is provided in Exhibit 5.1.

Session 1: Introduction and Overview

INTRODUCING MBTI: OVERVIEW AND EXPECTATIONS

During the first session of MBTI, it is very important to introduce the principles of mindfulness and metacognitive flexibility, demystify the practice of meditation, and provide expectations for the MBTI program. It is also important to establish ground rules for group discussions during each session, to emphasize the importance of establishing a home meditation practice, and to reinforce the concept of nonattachment to

EXHIBIT 5.1

MBTI Themes and Key Activities by Session

Session	Theme	Key activities
1	Introduction and overview of program	Provide overview of the program and participant expectations; introduce the concept of mindfulness and model of insomnia; lead participants through first formal mindful practice
2	Stepping out of automatic pilot	Begin with formal meditation and inquiry; discuss relevance of meditation for insomnia; discuss instructions for sleep hygiene
3	Paying attention to sleepiness and wakefulness	Begin with formal meditation and inquiry; discuss sleepiness, fatigue, and wakefulness; provide instructions for sleep consolidation
4	Working with sleeplessness at night	Begin with formal meditation and inquiry; discuss questions about sleep restriction and make adjustments to program; provide instructions for sleep reconditioning
5	The territory of insomnia	Begin with formal meditation and inquiry; introduce the territory of insomnia (both daytime and nighttime symptoms) and discuss this model
6	Acceptance and letting go	Begin with formal meditation and inquiry; explain the relevance of acceptance and letting go for working with thoughts and feelings in the territory of insomnia
7	Revisiting the relationship with sleep	Begin with formal meditation and inquiry; discuss participants' relationship with sleep (reactions to good and bad nights); discuss informal meditations during everyday life
8	Living mindfully after MBTI	Begin with formal meditation and inquiry; set up an action plan for future episodes of insomnia; discuss ways to continue mindfulness meditation beyond this program

Note. From "A Mindfulness-Based Approach to the Treatment of Insomnia," by J. Ong and D. Sholtes, 2010, *Journal of Clinical Psychology, 66,* p. 1179. Copyright 2010 by Wiley. Adapted with permission.

outcomes. Providing a syllabus can also give participants an idea of the upcoming schedule in terms of dates and content to be covered so that they can be clear about the expectations (see the Appendix for a sample syllabus). An outline for Session 1 is provided in Exhibit 5.2.

People often arrive at the first session hoping to improve their sleep quickly and permanently. This is understandable because many of these people have been suffering from insomnia for several years. One of the first concepts to communicate is that MBTI involves nonattachment to outcomes, including the attachment to better sleep. Participants are

EXHIBIT 5.2

Session 1 Outline

Theme: Introduction and Overview of the Program

Objectives
1. Provide an overview of the program and participant expectations.
2. Introduce the concept of mindfulness and initiate meditation practice.
3. Introduce the model of insomnia.

Activities
1. Introduction and Overview of the MBTI Program
    a. Distribute and review syllabus.
    b. Discuss ground rules and expectations.
    c. Provide group member introductions.

    Key Points: Provide participants with ground rules and expectations of the program. Introduce instructors and group members.

2. Meditation and Discussion
    a. Introduction to mindfulness meditation
    b. Mindful eating
    c. Inquiry and discussion of mindful eating
    d. Sitting meditation
    e. Introduce metaphors as needed (trainspotting, cloud meditation)

    Key Points: The raisin exercise is introduced as an example of how to eat mindfully and it can demonstrate how changes can take place by simply slowing down and paying attention to everyday activities. The sitting meditation provides participants with guidance on bringing attention to the breath. This serves as the anchor for grounding oneself in the present moment.

3. Insomnia Didactics and Strategies
    a. Discussion of 3-P model of insomnia

    Key Point: Introduce the model of insomnia that will be used in this program.

Homework for Session 1
1. Complete sleep and meditation diaries.
2. Eat at least one meal or snack mindfully each day.
3. Practice sitting with breath meditation for at least 15 minutes, at least 6 days during week.

instructed to set aside any goal or intention of trying to improve their sleep while they go through the program. MBTI instructors should pause for a moment to allow each participant the opportunity to let go of striving to make sleep better. Some participants will respond by asking why or expressing concern that this means they will have to give up on sleeping better. Others express pessimism and worry regarding what happens if MBTI does not work for them. In this context, a "healthy skepticism" is welcomed, but we encourage participants to remain open to "just do it" for now and to reevaluate their perspective at the end of the program. Sometimes it is helpful to discuss how previous participants began the program with similar levels of skepticism but were able to find success by the end of the program. Following are quotes from past participants in response to the question "If you were talking to someone who was considering this program, what advice would you give him or her?"

- "Come in with an open mind."
- "It is important to be committed."
- "Results depend on the effort you put into the program."
- "It's important to keep the meditation practices even when you are not seeing results—breakthroughs do happen!"

If necessary, MBTI instructors should explain that the purpose in letting go of trying to improve sleep will be discussed within the framework of mindfulness and self-compassion. At the end of the program, each participant will be given the opportunity to reevaluate his or her progress.

As part of the introduction, it is also important to create a safe space for participants to explore and discover their own journey in a mindful way. Instructors should establish ground rules for participants to follow during the group discussions. MBTI follows the approach taken in mindfulness-based stress reduction (MBSR), in which participants are instructed to refrain from giving advice to other members or making comments about how well one participant is doing, as this can be perceived as judgment that one member is doing better than another. Although offering advice can be tempting and might appear to be helpful at times, MBTI is not intended to be a support group for insomnia. Instead, this program teaches mindful listening, nonjudging, and being present without trying to engage in problem solving. During group discussions, the role of the MBTI instructor is to facilitate a dialogue on the discoveries and challenges that arise during meditations without trying to "teach" or engage in cognitive restructuring. This is a difficult skill that takes experience and practice to master and is aided by having a personal mindfulness meditation practice.

INTRODUCTION TO MINDFULNESS PRINCIPLES AND PRACTICES

For most participants, this will be their first formal training in mindfulness meditation. Some might have heard of mindfulness from a friend or read about it in a newspaper or magazine article, but most will be eager to learn what they will actually be doing. A good starting place is to begin by providing a historical background about mindfulness meditation, including its origins in Buddhism. This can also be a time to reinforce that mindfulness meditation is not taught as a religious practice in MBTI. Instead, these are principles grounded in Buddhist philosophy and science, which many people find are complementary with most religious beliefs. It is also important to explain that meditation practice is a central component of discovering mindfulness. In this discussion, it is often helpful to dispel myths regarding meditation. These include misconceptions that meditation is a special activity or that it promotes an altered state of consciousness. Quite the opposite is true—mindfulness meditation can be practiced in everyday activities and can create a clearer state of consciousness.

Next, the principles of mindfulness that are central to mindfulness-based therapies are discussed. These principles are identical to those used in MBSR (Kabat-Zinn, 1990) but are adapted in MBTI to include sleep-specific applications (see the Appendix, Handout 1). These principles or qualities are the core of adopting a mindful approach to each moment and can serve as guidelines for living in a mindful way. In MBTI, participants are asked to bring these principles into their daily lives by practicing the cultivation of mindfulness in their meditation practice. These principles are also used to begin teaching participants about metacognitions to enable them to make changes not only to the relationship with sleep, but also to sleep itself. These seven principles include the following:

- *Beginner's mind* involves the notion of approaching a situation or problem with a clear perspective that is not contingent upon past experiences, particularly negative past experiences. In the case of insomnia, many individuals feel that how they sleep the previous night will dictate how sleep will unfold this night, or they worry that every night will be the same.
- *Nonstriving.* During the course of insomnia, many people make increased efforts to sleep and forget that sleep is a process that cannot be forced but that, instead, should be allowed to unfold. Practicing the principle of nonstriving helps to maintain balance between the desire to sleep while allowing sleep to unfold.
- *Letting go.* Similar to nonstriving, attachment to the desire to make sleep happen or to achieve a certain amount of sleep tends to exacerbate the problem rather than make it better. Letting go is not the same as giving up—it involves intentionally letting go of the attachment to the problem rather than letting go of hope that the problem can be solved. Some MBSR instructors prefer the term *letting be* to emphasize that it is about allowing whatever is present to occur without automatically fixing it.
- *Nonjudging.* Most people are trained to analyze and judge problems in order to fix them. However, judgment can sometimes backfire and in the case of insomnia, automatically judging the state of being awake as negative and aversive can lead to negative energy, which can interfere with the process of sleep. Stepping back from

the problem and just observing it without judgment is one step towards metacognitive transformation.

- *Acceptance.* For many people, acceptance sounds like giving up and being at the mercy of insomnia. Much like letting go, acceptance does not imply that nothing can be done about the sleep problem, but rather that sleep cannot be directly controlled and that efforts to make it happen generally do not work. This is an active choice, allowing an opportunity to make value-congruent decisions. Some MBSR instructors prefer the term *acknowledgment* rather than acceptance because acknowledgement of what is present does not have the same negative connotation as acceptance.
- *Trust.* In the context of insomnia, trust involves a belief that our mind and body can self-regulate without interference. Knowledge about sleep physiology and the causes of insomnia can be helpful to cultivate confidence that "the brain isn't broken."
- *Patience.* Trusting sleep physiology to self-regulate also involves patience. Even if results do not happen immediately (and they usually do take time), patience in the process, as opposed to the outcome, reduces the sleep-related anxiety and the tendency to be reactive.

MBTI instructors should note that many of these principles will not be easy to implement immediately. Letting go and acceptance tend to be particularly challenging principles to acquire, and most individuals new to the practice of mindfulness will not be ready to skillfully apply these principles to work with their symptoms of insomnia. In this early phase of MBTI, instructors should provide a clear explanation of each principle and encourage participants to see how these principles might fit into their lives. A more thorough discussion on acceptance and letting go will occur later in MBTI after participants have had a chance to engage in a few weeks of meditation practice (see Chapter 7).

After describing the background and principles of mindfulness, it is time to begin practicing meditation. In choosing the first meditation, MBTI instructors should select a regular activity that can be done in a mindful way. This helps to demystify some misconceptions of meditation and also provides an opportunity to discuss how mindfulness can be integrated into daily activities. Following the tradition established in MBSR, the mindful eating exercise can serve as an excellent first meditation in MBTI. This exercise is introduced as an example of how to eat mindfully, and it can demonstrate how we are often unaware of what is going on in our normal everyday activities. It can also demonstrate how changes can take place by simply slowing down and paying attention to these activities rather than changing the activities themselves. This exercise also provides an example of how mindfulness practice does not have to be just a formal sitting meditation. See Exhibit 5.3 for guidance on leading a mindful eating exercise.

EXHIBIT 5.3

Mindful Eating

Notes: The following exercise is completed in about 10 minutes to serve as a first experience of mindfulness meditation. Instructors should guide the participant to eat each piece of food (e.g., raisin) in a mindful way using each of the senses in a very deliberate manner.

Instructions:
1. Select a food that is common and relatively small. Raisins or nuts are excellent choices. Instruct each participant to take two or three pieces of the food, setting the food in front of them.
2. Guide participants to slowly use each of their senses to experience the food. Begin with the sense of sight by telling participants to look at the food, noticing things such as color, texture, shininess, and so forth. Next, ask participants to touch the food using one finger, again noticing any sensations such as texture, sliminess, smoothness, or roughness. Then, have participants hold the object up to their ear and listen to the food. Sometimes, people giggle about this, as it seems silly to "listen to food." If there is no sound or noise, that's fine—it's a reminder that we can pay attention to silence or absence of sensation. Then, ask participants to bring the object to the nose and smell it, noticing any aromas or odors (positive or negative). Finally, tell participants to put the object in their mouth. First, ask them to notice if there is an automatic tendency to swallow when an object is put inside the mouth. Second, ask participants to bring awareness to the flavors in the mouth, noticing where those flavors are occurring on the tongue (different flavors are picked up by different parts of the tongue). Finally, ask participants to swallow the object and reflect upon the process of eating.
3. After a moment of reflection, instruct participants to eat the remaining food on their own in the same way described above. Instructors can also engage in mindful eating with the participants, or observe participants as they are engaging in the activity.
4. If needed, encourage participants to pay attention to thoughts about the raisin—liking or disliking the raisin; judgments about smell, taste, texture, and so forth.
5. This exercise is processed and contrasted with the normal eating experience. Furthermore, it is offered as an example of how mindfulness can apply to common activities in their lives to demystify the concept that it is a special activity.

After guiding participants through the mindful eating meditation, the MBTI instructor facilitates a period of inquiry and discussion to allow participants to process this experience. Often, participants will comment that they feel "silly" or make a statement that reflects immediate judgment, such as "raisins are gross." It is important for the MBTI instructor to embody the principle of nonjudging and to allow participants to voice their discoveries rather than trying to get them to "say the right thing." Instructors can note the tendency of the mind to automatically assign positive and negative qualities (e.g., "This reminds me how much I hate raisins"), but instructors should refrain from engaging in any kind of cognitive restructuring, such as correcting a thought and replacing it with another thought or showing preference for a positive thought. This encourages participants to openly share their reactions without editing, an important first step in cultivating awareness.

Following this informal meditation, participants are introduced to their first formal sitting meditation. This meditation focuses on the breath and describes how sitting and observing the process of breathing serve as a foundational meditation that other meditations can build upon. One important message to convey is that breathing is a physiological activity that can be automatically controlled by the brain or brought under conscious control. We do not have to think about breathing in order to do it, but we have the ability to breathe in certain intentional ways, and we can bring our active attention to the process of breathing to guide it. In this first breathing meditation, participants are encouraged to bring awareness to the sensations that are created by observing this process, noting physical sensations, changes in muscle tension, tickling of the nostrils, or other sensations. Sometimes participants will comment about not doing it right, but as long as they are bringing their awareness to what is occurring in the moment and are able to describe these sensations, then they are practicing mindfulness. The first key point to mindfulness meditation is that as long as you are intentionally bringing your awareness to the process, there is no wrong way to meditate! Typically, the first guided sitting meditation lasts 10 to 15 minutes, followed by a period of inquiry and discussion. See Exhibit 5.4 for guidance on leading a sitting meditation.

In addition to the formal meditations, metaphors can serve as a useful illustration for participants who find that activities like focusing on the breath or "watching things rise and fall in the mind" are too vague or unstructured. For example, the *trainspotting metaphor* (see Exhibit 5.5) illustrates how thoughts come in and out of the mind like trains passing through a station. In this metaphor, most of us are used to being passengers, carried from station to station on the train, just like how we typically "ride" inside our thoughts. These thoughts then carry us from place to place, often without our awareness of where they are taking us. In contrast, mindful awareness allows us to decenter from the thoughts and observe them as mental activities. In the metaphor, trainspotters are people who enjoy observing trains go by because of a curiosity and interest in the train itself. They are not using trains as a form of transportation, but they instead observe the qualities of each train—the type of train, how fast it is going, and how full it is—with an interest in the train itself, not its destination. Much like being a passenger and stepping off the train onto the platform and watching from there as trains go by, it is possible to just watch thoughts go by in the mind without following them to their destination. This is a metacognitive shift from an outcome-oriented mode (i.e., thoughts that lead to problem solving) to a process-oriented mode (i.e., observing the thoughts themselves). Instructors can use the

EXHIBIT 5.4

Sitting Meditation

Notes: This meditation can be done while seated in chairs or sitting on the ground. For the first meditation, instructors should provide more details to participants to guide them through the process of bringing attention to the breath. In later MBTI sessions, instructors can transition to providing less guidance and allow participants more space to explore. Typical duration is 20 to 30 minutes.

Instructions:
1. Begin by having participants sit in a comfortable position (in a chair or on the ground), bringing awareness to their posture.
2. Have participants close their eyes. They may also do this meditation with the eyes open.
3. Take a moment to welcome participants into this space and begin to take note of any thoughts, feelings, and sensations in this moment.
4. On the next inhalation, have participants take a slow, deep breath, paying particular attention to the sensations in the body that arise during the process of inhalation. This might include noticing the belly move, the chest expand, or the movement of air into the nostrils.
5. On the exhalation, tell participants to slowly let out the air from the nose or mouth, again paying particular attention to the sensations in the body that arise during the process of exhalation. This might include the belly sinking, the shoulders dropping, or the air moving out of the nostrils or mouth.
6. With each breath, remind participants to bring full awareness to the process of breathing. Notice the sensations in the body as the air moves in and out.
7. Ask participants to find a particular location, such as the mouth, nostrils, or belly, and focus on sensations in that particular region of the body as they continue to breathe in and out. Allow participants space to explore sensations on their own for a period of time.
8. After a few minutes, mindfully check in with participants and ask them to notice if their mind has wandered. Acknowledge that the mind has a tendency to wander and if this happens, they have not done anything wrong. Simply bring awareness to mind wandering and gently and with compassion, bring attention back to the breath.
9. Instructors can expand awareness from the breath to include the body, sounds in the environment, sounds within the body, and thoughts in the mind.
10. If awareness has been expanded, bring the focus of attention back to the breath for a few minutes.
11. End the meditation by ringing the chimes or bell.

trainspotting metaphor to explain how to disengage and watch thoughts. Furthermore, "stepping off the train" and "becoming a trainspotter" can be useful phrases for participants to use in their training to observe thoughts without attachment to outcomes.

The *cloud metaphor* can be another useful way to explain mindfulness principles. The purpose of this activity is to watch thoughts as if they were clouds in the sky. It can serve as a metaphor for the futility of trying to control thoughts or to prevent certain thoughts from happening. Similar to the trainspotting metaphor, the cloud metaphor provides an opportunity to practice observing thoughts without engaging in the

EXHIBIT 5.5

Trainspotting Metaphor

Notes: The trainspotting metaphor is used as a way to illustrate the difference between observing thoughts as they arise in the mind and becoming engaged in thoughts. Although not a formal meditation, it can be explained as a metaphor alone or it can be delivered as part of a sitting meditation where the focus is on watching thoughts in the mind.

Instructions for using trainspotting in a meditation:
1. Ask participants to lie down or sit in a relaxed position and close their eyes, then take a few slow, deep breaths, bringing full awareness to the breath.
2. Slowly ask participants to bring attention away from the outside world and into the mind, imagining that they are standing on the platform of a train station. Ask them to look around this train station and imagine their thoughts as trains, racing by the station one at a time.
3. Encourage participants to observe each thought, whatever comes to mind. There are no right thoughts or wrong thoughts; some might be fast-moving and some might be slower lumbering ones. Rather than focusing on the thought and thinking about where it will lead (i.e., getting on the train), remind participants to stand back and observe the thought. It might be helpful to offer a few prompts, such as: *Where did it come from? Is it positive or negative? Where is it going?*
4. Provide guidance to acknowledge that the mind is likely to engage in the thought or "jump on a train" in the metaphor. Remind participants to notice when they have "stepped on a train" and to gently bring themselves back to the platform. Encourage the practice of self-compassion by acknowledging that this is okay and simply return to trainspotting on the platform. Also note that participants should continue to go through the same process each time they notice that they are no longer trainspotting.
5. Instruct the participant to bring the attention back to the breath. Close the meditation by ringing the chimes or a bell.
6. After the meditation is completed, remind participants that it takes practice to be a trainspotter. Encourage them to practice trainspotting, formally or informally, to see if there is a metacognitive shift in perspective.

process of interpreting or acting on the thoughts. It is also seen as promoting the metacognitive skill of decentering from the thoughts, such that thoughts can be thoughts without judgment or attachment to achieving an outcome. Using weather as part of the metaphor, thoughts in the mind are seen as clouds rolling by during the day. By watching clouds closely, one will notice that they come and go. Sometimes they hover around for longer periods; other times they pass quickly. One might also notice that weather is always changing and we do not have control over it. Watching clouds can give us an indication of what the weather will be like and help us prepare, but there is nothing we can do to change the weather. It is also possible to use the cloud metaphor as part of a guided meditation to help participants observe thoughts. Exhibit 5.6 provides instructions for delivering the cloud metaphor as part of a meditation.

EXHIBIT 5.6

Cloud Metaphor

Notes: The cloud metaphor serves to demonstrate how futile it is to try and control thoughts or to prevent certain thoughts from happening. Similar to the trainspotting metaphor, this can be explained as a metaphor, or it can be used as part of a sitting meditation where the focus is on thoughts.

Instructions for using the clouds in a meditation:
1. Ask participants to lie down or sit in a relaxed position and close their eyes, then take a few slow, deep breaths, bringing full awareness to the breath.
2. Ask participants to slowly bring attention away from the outside world and into the mind, imagining that they are looking up at the sky. Ask them to imagine that their thoughts are clouds, floating around the sky.
3. Instruct participants to just observe the clouds, noticing the color, shape, and type of cloud. Some clouds might be white and fluffy, while other clouds might be gray. Sometimes clouds will blow away quickly, while other clouds will stay around longer. Remind participants to just observe the clouds rather than analyze what they might mean or what they might bring.
4. Introduce the idea that observing clouds for a period of time can sometimes lead us to recognize patterns. In this way, thoughts might indicate a particular theme or struggle we are having. If this occurs, just make note of it. Remind participants that this activity is not meant to solve problems but simply to "observe weather patterns." Mindful action can be taken after the meditation.
5. Instruct participants to bring the attention back to the breath. Close the meditation by ringing the chimes or bell.
6. After the meditation is completed, the period of inquiry can include a discussion of the "weather patterns" that were observed. It might be helpful to discuss how clouds can sometimes provide an indication of a change in the weather or a storm, which is symbolic of emotional distress. This could point towards an unresolved conflict or stress that needs to be addressed. This can be discussed as an example of how mindful awareness can help lead to mindful action.

INSTRUCTIONS FOR LEADING GUIDED MEDITATIONS

Leading guided meditations takes experience, and a personal meditation practice is extremely helpful. Instructors should keep a few important points in mind when leading guided meditations. First, MBTI instructors should be practicing mindfulness principles as they are guiding the meditation rather than reading from a script. It is important to embody the mindfulness principles and to enhance the authenticity of whatever is arising in the moment for the MBTI instructors. As such, instructors should be aware of the volume of their voice, making sure that all participants can hear them. Second, it is important to use simple language and present participles (i.e., verbs ending in *ing*). The choice of the present participle reinforces the present-moment attention of the meditation, and simple language is preferred so that participants do not have to process the instructions. In addition, it is important for instructors to provide space by pausing between instructions during the meditations to allow participants to register the experience and discover what is arising in that moment. The pace of the meditation should be moderate, with sufficient time between instructions to allow participants to explore, but not so long that participants get lost in terms of what they should be doing. It might be helpful to offer more guidance during the initial meditations and less as the program progresses and participants become more accustomed to the meditations.

Following a guided meditation, almost every participant will comment at some point that his or her mind is wandering and/or he or she is having difficulty maintaining focus throughout the entire meditation. It is vital that MBTI instructors communicate the universality of mind wandering and normalize this as something to expect during meditations. Instructors can provide guidance to participants by instructing them to note that wandering has occurred or that distraction is present and to gently redirect attention back to the object of interest, such as the sensations of breathing. In doing so, instructors can reinforce the fact that there is no "right way" or "wrong way" to meditate and there is no preference for eliminating mind wandering during the meditation. They should clearly communicate the concept of nonjudgmental acceptance early in the program. Following other meditation traditions, the meditations in MBTI usually conclude with the ringing of the bells or chimes.

INTRODUCING INSOMNIA AS A 24-HOUR PROBLEM

MBTI is built on the concept that insomnia is a 24-hour problem, not just a problem at night. Recall from Chapter 1 that the 3-P model of insomnia (Spielman, Caruso, & Glovinsky, 1987) has been very influential in the conceptualization of insomnia. As a reminder, the 3-P model explains the development and maintenance of insomnia as involving predisposing, precipitating, and perpetuating factors. This model is very useful because it applies the diathesis–stress model, one of the most influential models that describe the impact of stress on the body, to the known mechanisms of sleep and wakefulness. Furthermore, the novelty of the perpetuating factor highlights the role that reacting to sleep disturbance and increasing sleep effort plays in the etiology of insomnia. The perpetuation of insomnia is therefore driven by an elevation in arousal or hyperarousal that is prominent in individuals with chronic insomnia (Bonnet & Arand, 2010; Riemann et al., 2010). When people with insomnia are in a state of hyperarousal, they feel as if they are constantly "tired but wired" and have difficulty relaxing or letting go of wakefulness, even though they desperately want to be sleeping. For example, some people with insomnia have described their bed as "an enemy" or the bedtime as a "battlefield" and if they lose this "battle" they have to pay the consequences the next day. Others have spent so much time trying to fix their sleep problem that they spend more waking hours thinking about sleep than actually getting sleep.

Explaining the 3-P model to patients in the first session is important because it provides a clear understanding of what contributes to chronic insomnia and why it is different from the occasional sleep disturbances that everyone experiences. The explanation also provides hope that there are factors that can be directly addressed even though sleep cannot be directly increased. Specifically, the model helps participants understand that who they are (i.e., predisposing factors) might contribute to their likelihood of developing insomnia and that stress is likely to trigger sleep disturbance (i.e., precipitating factor). However, it is the reaction and increased effort of trying to obtain sleep (i.e., perpetuating factor) that causes a state of hyperarousal and leads to the vicious cycle of chronic insomnia. Fortunately, it is possible to address the reactivity and effort to sleep, which is why MBTI approaches insomnia as a 24-hour problem, not just a matter of what happens at night. The 3-P model also serves to prime participants to think differently about their insomnia symptoms, which will eventually feed into the concept of the territory of insomnia, discussed later in MBTI.

HOMEWORK FOR SESSION 1

In wrapping up the first session, it is important to communicate expectations for patients to engage in homework to practice the principles of mindfulness and digest the concepts of insomnia. Typically, the homework assignments will involve meditation practices, along with some instructions about making changes in sleep-related activities. Instructors might also include supplemental reading materials about mindfulness and insomnia, such as book chapters or articles.

Meditation Practice

For Session 1, the primary goal is for participants to begin practicing meditation on their own and to figure out when, where, and how they will establish a meditation practice. Rather than giving specific instructions or guidelines about these parameters, instructors should encourage participants to try practicing at different times and places so that they can discover for themselves what works. Inevitably, a few participants in each group will encounter challenges. Rather than viewing this as a negative, instructors can use it as an opportunity in Session 2 to discuss the ubiquitous nature of these challenges and to promote a sense of group camaraderie in practicing mindfulness meditation.

For homework, participants should eat at least one meal or snack mindfully each day, so that they can apply the qualities of mindfulness to a common daily activity. Participants should also practice the sitting meditation for at least 15 minutes, at least 6 days during the upcoming week. There is no special reason for the number or duration of meditation. These instructions were generally adopted from the MBSR and mindfulness-based cognitive therapy programs along with my personal observations as to what was feasible for most participants. Instructors should feel free to make adjustments on the basis of their experience or the characteristics of the participants in the group. A meditation diary should also be provided so that participants can keep track of the number of meditations, duration of each meditation session, and type of meditation (see the Appendix for an example).

Sleep Diaries

In addition to the meditation diaries, having participants keep sleep diaries is an important self-monitoring tool in MBTI. During the first session, it is important to explain how monitoring sleep is a fundamental tool that is used to cultivate awareness of sleep and daytime patterns across days and nights. Completing prospective diaries (as opposed to retrospective recall) is an important method to examine sleep-related behaviors and to monitor changes in sleep over time. Sleep diaries provide important information for the patient to develop greater awareness of sleep–wake patterns and sleep-related behaviors. MBTI instructors and researchers can use them to assess progress and outcomes of patients who complete MBTI. Later in MBTI, the information from the sleep diaries will be used to set schedules of when to go to bed and when to get out of bed (see Chapter 6).

Sleep diaries can take many forms, and each has certain advantages and disadvantages. Recently, a standardized sleep diary was published that contains instructions for completing the diary, and a core and extended version that can be used for gathering additional data (Carney et al., 2012). The key sleep–wake parameters that should be collected for MBTI include lights out (i.e., time going to bed at night), sleep onset latency (SOL), number of awakenings (NWAK), wake after sleep onset (WASO), early morning awakenings (EMA), lights on (i.e., time getting up in the morning), and a rating of sleep quality. From these parameters, total wake time (TWT), total sleep time (TST), and sleep efficiency (SE) can be calculated. In addition to these nighttime parameters, ratings of daytime sleepiness/alertness and fatigue/energy can be useful in assessing changes in daytime functioning. Instructors should take time to review the sleep diaries and make sure that participants understand their purpose and the instructions. Although the standardized sleep diary can serve as a helpful starting point, MBTI instructors should make adaptations or additions as needed. Derivation of the sleep parameters and the use of these data in implementing specific behavioral techniques are discussed later in Chapter 6. Handout 3 in the Appendix is an example of a sleep diary.

Session 2: Stepping Out of Automatic Pilot

The theme for Session 2 is *stepping out of automatic pilot,* which refers to the concept of experiencing the present moment fully and intentionally, not just going through the motions. Building on the introduction to the concepts and practices of mindfulness in Session 1, Session 2 focuses on establishing and deepening the meditation practice with an emphasis on cultivating awareness and intention of the thoughts, feelings, and sensations that arise in the present moment. This practice is the platform that is needed to step out of automatic pilot. As part of this theme, the behavioral instructions for sleep hygiene are introduced and reviewed with participants. See Exhibit 5.7 for the Session 2 outline.

The typical structure of the MBTI session also begins to take shape in Session 2. The first hour is spent on two guided meditations (20–30 minutes each), followed by a period of inquiry and discussion (10–15 minutes). The period of inquiry serves as a time and space for discussing the meditation practices in class, discoveries during the meditation practice at home, and the application of mindfulness principles in the lives of the participants. Instructions for leading this period are provided in the following paragraphs. After a short 10- to 15-minute break, the remaining hour is spent on didactics or instructions related to insomnia. These include behavioral strategies and metacognitive strategies that will be discussed later in this chapter and in Chapters 6 and 7.

OPENING MEDITATION PRACTICE AND PERIOD OF INQUIRY AND DISCUSSION

To help establish the structure of opening each session with meditation practice, instructors should begin Session 2 with a 20- to 30-minute sitting meditation practice (see Exhibit 5.4). This meditation was introduced during Session 1, and opening Session 2 with it can remind participants of this foundational practice and deepen the experience of mindfulness by extending the duration of the meditation. During this practice, instruc-

EXHIBIT 5.7

Session 2 Outline

Theme: Stepping Out of Automatic Pilot

Objectives
1. Establish each participant's own meditation practice.
2. Explain how to step out of automatic pilot and bring awareness to the mind and body.
3. Provide instructions for sleep hygiene.

Activities
1. Meditation Practice and Inquiry
   a. Sitting meditation
   b. Body scan meditation

   Key Point: The sitting and body scan meditations serve as a means of stepping out of automatic pilot (i.e., being unaware of habitual physical or emotional reactive patterns) by bringing intentional awareness to the breath and specific body areas.

2. Insomnia Didactics and Strategies
   a. Discussion of sleep hygiene

   Key Point: Discuss sleep hygiene as a way to notice any behaviors or activities that might be incompatible with sleep. Bring awareness to the things that we do (or don't do) to facilitate sleep.

Homework for Session 2
1. Complete sleep and meditation diaries.
2. Practice body scan meditation using CD (30 minutes each session for at least 6 days).
3. Follow sleep hygiene instructions throughout this week.

tors should carefully and gently guide participants, remembering to create a safe space and also to emphasize that there is no right or wrong way to meditate. After completing the sitting meditation practice, the instructor should lead a period of inquiry and discussion. The period of inquiry follows a Buddhist tradition whereby students have an opportunity to openly ask questions and discuss their experiences with the meditation practice. The first line of inquiry is on the meditation that was just completed. The instructor can open the dialogue by asking participants what they noticed during the meditation practice. Participants should be encouraged to maintain mindfulness principles during this period of inquiry by describing any experience that came up during the meditation in a nonjudgmental manner. It does not have to be an interesting or profound experience, and the instructor should be careful how they respond to the participants' experiences. The instructor's job is not to tell students what they should be experiencing or learning, but to gently guide them to observe their own experiences and to listen mindfully to those of others. Instructors can highlight what they are hearing from participants, but they should avoid judging whether

an experience is good or bad or expressing more interest when participants report more radical experiences. This takes mindful practice on
the instructor's part. For instructors who might be trained as CBT therapists, it can be very tempting to fall into the trap of teaching. However,
in MBTI the meditation practice is the primary teacher.

The second line of inquiry should be aimed at the connection between
the meditation practice at home and overall well-being. This includes
noticing any changes in the symptoms of insomnia, daytime functioning,
or other areas related to the quality of life. This can be a time to review
the homework assignment for meditation practice and for participants to
discuss what they discovered in their home meditation practice. In the
second session, participants will have had only 1 week to begin establishing a meditation practice, and almost every participant will report
difficulties and challenges in establishing the practice. Comments usually
include lack of time, space, privacy, or difficulties in keeping the mind
focused. These challenges should be acknowledged, and participants
should be encouraged to continue with their commitment to establishing
a meditation practice and see how they might find creative solutions to
work with these challenges. If needed, it can be helpful here to remind
participants of the principles and concepts of mindfulness practice. It is
quite common that in the discussion one participant might describe a
solution that another person had not yet considered, and therefore the
group as a whole benefits from the discussion. This is one of the reasons
behind having a period of inquiry in a group format.

BODY SCAN MEDITATION

Following the period of inquiry and discussion, a second formal meditation is introduced: the *body scan*. The body scan meditation serves as an
important exercise for intentionally bringing awareness to a particular
body area, noting sensations without trying to alter or change anything,
and then letting go and bringing attention to another part of the body.
This meditation also emphasizes the point of stepping out of a mindless
mode in which one is unaware of the habitual physical or emotional
reactive patterns. Specifically, the body scan meditation deepens the connection with the body as we become more aware of each part of the
body. This is particularly important for certain areas that do not typically
receive conscious attention, such as the bottom of the feet or the top of
the head. Because the body scan meditation lasts for about 30 minutes,
it also helps participants to practice sustained, focused attention over
a period of time and to learn how to redirect attention back to the
body when attention has wandered. This practice of attention and intention is vital to the practice of mindfulness meditation. The body scan is
introduced as an exercise in awareness, in which participants direct their

attention toward whatever they are experiencing in the body while they are reminded to maintain a gentle, nonjudgmental awareness throughout the meditation.

In addition to physical awareness, the body scan also serves to develop awareness of emotions and can lead to a sense of calmness, or equanimity. It provides an opportunity to practice bringing a gentle, curious awareness to sensations in the body as they arise in the present moment. A greater awareness of the body is important in learning how to deal more effectively with emotions. Specific sensations such as tightness in the chest or tension in the shoulders may at times signal the presence of strong feelings that are somaticized and not experienced with conscious awareness. Feedback on how the body feels is an integral part of learning how to better manage emotions and stress.

MBTI instructors should note that although the body scan provides an opportunity to enter into a deep state of physical and mental relaxation, instructors should make it clear that this meditation practice is not intended to directly help participants fall asleep. It might be helpful to remind participants that the intention is not to "meditate yourself to sleep" but instead to use this exercise to cultivate awareness. Although the body scan might eventually help participants fall asleep, it is important that they learn to practice how to cultivate awareness of the body sensations without using it to try to help their insomnia. After mastering this skill through practice, the body scan can then be used to facilitate sleepiness at night. If participants happen to fall asleep unintentionally, MBTI instructors should still practice nonjudgment so that participants do not feel guilty about falling asleep. If this occurs, instructors can gently awaken the participant after the body scan meditation is completed. This can sometimes provide an opportunity to discuss how sleep can emerge when sleep effort is reduced. See Exhibit 5.8 for instruction on leading the body scan meditation.

As with the sitting meditation, a period of inquiry and discussion should follow to promote dialogue on the participant's initial experience with the body scan. Some participants report a sense of relaxation or sleepiness, whereas others describe restlessness. Most participants say that it is difficult or annoying to progress so slowly from one body part to another. Again, the instructor should reinforce the principles of mindfulness and explain how this practice is an important means of getting out of the rushed, problem-solving mode and into a more patient, mindful mode. To promote the dialogue, instructors might ask one or more of the following questions:

1. Did you notice anything different about your body?
2. Did anyone fall asleep?
3. How do you think the body scan will help you to work with insomnia?

EXHIBIT 5.8

Body Scan Meditation

Notes: The body scan meditation is an important meditation for practicing how to intentionally bring awareness to a particular body area, noting sensations without trying to alter or change anything, and then letting go and bringing attention to another part of the body. This meditation should be done by having participants lie on yoga mats. The lights can be dimmed if desired. Although the body scan provides an opportunity to enter into a deep state of physical and mental relaxation, instructors should make it clear that this practice is not intended to help people fall asleep. The body scan typically lasts for about 30 minutes.

Instructions:
1. Have participants lie down with their eyes closed.
2. Take a moment to welcome participants into this space and begin to take note of any thoughts, feelings, and sensations in this moment.
3. Bring awareness to the breath by taking a slow, deep, breath, paying particular attention to the sensations in the body that arise during the inhalation and during the exhalation. This might include noticing the belly move, the chest expand, or the movement of air into the nostrils.
4. After bringing mindful awareness to a few breaths, prepare participants for the body scan by instructing them to pay attention to any physical sensations that arise, such as itchiness, tension, tightness, pain, or neutrality. If pain or tightness is present, encourage participants to allow it to release or let go. If that is not possible, try bringing awareness to the sensation of pain rather than making it go away.
5. Begin the body scan with the left foot. Bring full awareness to this part of the body, noting all of the sensations that are present without judgment. Allow participants to explore for about 1 to 2 minutes.
6. After taking a mindful breath, allow the awareness to withdraw from the left foot and move it to the left ankle and lower leg. Again, bring full awareness to this part of the body, noting all of the sensations that are present without judgment. Allow participants to explore for about 1 to 2 minutes.
7. Guide participants through each part of the body, moving up from the lower left leg to the upper left leg, then shifting to the right foot and then up the leg. From there, move to the back, the torso, shoulders, each arm, and finally ending at the head.
8. Periodically, check in with the participants about mind wandering. If the attention wanders, participants are encouraged to note that their mind has wandered and to gently bring attention back to the part of the body being scanned. This is in contrast to forcing attention or clearing the mind.
9. After bringing awareness to the head, awareness should be brought to the body as a whole, noticing the connection between the different parts of the body.
10. Bring the awareness back to the breath, for one or two breaths.
11. End the meditation by ringing the chimes or bell.

These questions are designed to help participants draw connections between the mindful stance that is cultivated during a meditation practice and how this mindful stance can help them work with the symptoms of insomnia. As participants begin to understand the principles of mindfulness and to report discoveries of metacognitive shifts during their practice, the MBTI instructor might ask the third question to help participants consider the opportunity to practice these shifts when insomnia symptoms are present. Although this question might appear to promote outcome-oriented thinking, it can actually start a discussion about the balance of being mindful and experiencing the symptoms of insomnia. Also, participants should be reminded that the cause of suffering is the attachment to outcomes, not the acknowledgment of outcomes. Suppressing thoughts of wanting to sleep better is not the same thing as letting go of those thoughts. A mindful stance does not entail avoidance of the outcome; instead, it is about letting go of it as a thought. Here instructors might want to remind participants about the principle of letting go and note that Session 6 includes a more thorough discussion of applying the principle of letting go to work with sleep-related thoughts (see Chapter 7).

WHY IS AWARENESS IMPORTANT
FOR WORKING WITH INSOMNIA?

At this point in the MBTI program, participants will have experienced two of the foundational meditations. They should also have begun to practice meditation at home. With a taste of what MBTI is about, it is fairly common for participants to begin wondering how their efforts to meditate will directly apply to resolving their insomnia disorder, especially if they have not seen any changes yet. The insomnia-related didactics for Session 2 begin by addressing this question. The goal is to provide participants with a rationale for the connection between developing awareness through mindfulness meditation and its potential impact on insomnia. This is another chance to emphasize how habitual reactions to sleep and sleeplessness contribute to the problem of insomnia.

Rather than providing specific guidelines for leading this didactic, MBTI instructors should develop their own style and deliver the message using examples from the group discussions or their previous experience. In doing so, there are two key points to make in explaining this connection to the participants. First, the automatic pilot in the context of insomnia involves automatic tendencies, habits, or thoughts that tend to occur as a reaction to sleep disturbance. For example, if one feels fatigued or sleepy the next day, the blame might be put automatically on the previous night's sleep. Or one might feel that if 7 hours of sleep are not achieved, then the next-day functioning will be automatically suboptimal. Other tendencies might be seen in compensation, such as resetting the alarm clock for a later time to make up for lost sleep, drinking more coffee during the day, or trying to fall asleep whenever possible. Here, it is important to help patients make specific connections with what types of thoughts and behaviors to be aware of in the context of insomnia. The second key point is that the awareness of these reactions serves as the platform for taking mindful action. This is important because it is the first step in shifting from a mindless, reactive stance to a more intentional, active, and mindful stance. Without intentional, present-moment awareness, it is very difficult to make metacognitive or behavioral changes related to improving symptoms of insomnia.

SLEEP HYGIENE

In addition to helping patients make specific connections between the concept of awareness and the context of insomnia, sleep hygiene recommendations are presented as a way to bring awareness to behaviors or activities that might be incompatible with sleep. Many people have heard the term *sleep hygiene*, but this term has become overused by the media and by health care providers. Stepanski and Wyatt (2003) reviewed the literature on sleep hygiene and found that (a) there was variability in what recommendations were included under the term *sleep hygiene* and (b) when the original recommendations of sleep hygiene were tested, it had only a small effect on improving sleep when administered as a lone intervention. Therefore, in the context of MBTI, sleep hygiene is recommended as a first step in developing awareness of sleep-related habits and behaviors. It is not expected that following good sleep hygiene alone will have a strong impact for most individuals with chronic insomnia. The main components of sleep hygiene are listed as follows (see Handout 4 in the Appendix):

- Be aware of the timing and amount of time spent in bed. Regularize the timing and amount of time in bed.
- Be aware of sleep effort. Avoid putting effort into trying to sleep.
- Monitor intake of substances. Avoid coffee, alcohol, and nicotine starting from the late afternoon or evening.
- Regular, moderate exercise can promote sleep over the long run, but attempts to use exercise to "tire oneself to sleep" are not effective.
- Monitor eating habits by avoiding late meals. However, a light snack at bedtime is not likely to have a negative impact on sleep.
- Manage the environment in terms of noise, temperature, comfort, and safety.

Participants might remark that these recommendations are general, rather than specific. Much like good dental hygiene is a way to promote healthy teeth and reduce the risk of having cavities, sleep hygiene is a way to promote awareness of sleep-related behaviors in order to reduce the risk of having trouble falling or staying asleep. Instructors should caution participants that, in itself, following sleep hygiene recommendations can reduce the risk of poor sleep but might not immediately improve sleep. Also, many patients will comment that these recommendations sound familiar, and they might have even tried using them with limited success. If that is the case, the instructor can gently acknowledge these past attempts but encourage participants to practice beginner's mind and to either continue following these rules or try again, regardless of the previous outcome.

When introducing sleep hygiene, MBTI instructors can distribute and review a handout for sleep hygiene instructions and review this with the group (see the Appendix, Handout 4). They should be prepared to discuss the application of these instructions consistently and explain how these instructions are only part of the program. This can also be a good time to review the sleep diaries with the participants and to discuss any discoveries they might have had about their sleep patterns over the past week. Again, some participants might express frustration that no improvements have occurred as of yet. MBTI instructors should acknowledge this frustration and provide gentle encouragement to continue the practice and activities in the MBTI program and to be open to discoveries other than to the attachment to sleep improvement.

HOMEWORK FOR SESSION 2

The homework assignment for Session 2 is to continue the meditation and sleep diaries. For the meditation practice, participants are asked to practice the body scan meditation using guidance from digital media (e.g., CD or electronic file) for at least 6 days. For sleep recommendations, participants are asked to practice the sleep hygiene recommendations and to report any discoveries about their experience in implementing these instructions. At this point, participants should have a solid foundation of the conceptual basis of MBTI and the practice of formal meditation. With an understanding of the importance of cultivating awareness as the first step, participants are now set for the next phase of MBTI—using mindful awareness to make wise choices when sleep disturbance and hyperarousal are present.

Reprogramming the Brain for Sleep

6

T he first two sessions of mindfulness-based therapy for insomnia (MBTI) build the foundation for cultivating present-moment awareness through meditation practice. In Sessions 3 and 4, participants are taught how to use awareness of mental and physical states to make sleep-related decisions that are intentional and mindful. At the crux of this is the recognition of thoughts, feelings, and physical sensations that can discern the state of sleepiness from other states, such as fatigue. By identifying the sensations associated with sleepiness, patients are able to connect with the signals from the brain indicating readiness for sleep. With a clearer indication of sleepiness, patients are provided with instructions for managing sleep-related behaviors on the basis of the state of sleepiness, allowing them to increase the likelihood that sleep will occur when they are in bed. These instructions usually differ from how patients have previously reacted to the sensations of sleepiness and fatigue. In this manner, patients are "reprogramming the brain for sleep."

http://dx.doi.org/10.1037/14952-007

Mindfulness-Based Therapy for Insomnia, by J. C. Ong

Sessions 3 and 4 also offer a progression of formal meditations to include awareness of the body in motion, providing an opportunity to deepen and expand the meditation practice. Quiet meditations serve as the starting point for practicing mindfulness and include the sitting meditation, breathing meditation, and body scan described in Chapter 5. As the MBTI program moves into the third and fourth classes, the types of meditations are expanded to include movement meditations. Walking meditations and mindful stretching, or light hatha yoga, are the movement meditations that are typically introduced. Some instructors who have experience with tai chi or qi gong might feel comfortable incorporating these techniques, as long as the principles of mindfulness are kept in mind. The purpose of the movement meditations is to extend the practice of mindful awareness while the body is still into the practice of mindful awareness while the body is in motion. By beginning with awareness of the breath, moving to a sitting meditation and then the body scan, and extending to a walking meditation or yoga, the field of mindful awareness is progressively expanded. Later, informal meditations are reintroduced, further expanding the practice to mindful awareness during everyday activities such as eating, exercising, working, and relating to family members.

In Session 3, the walking meditation is introduced and instructions for sleep consolidation are provided. In MBTI, sleep consolidation is an adaption of sleep restriction therapy (Spielman, Saskin, & Thorpy, 1987) using mindfulness principles. In Session 4, mindful stretching and light yoga are introduced along with instructions for sleep reconditioning. In MBTI, sleep reconditioning is an adaption of stimulus control instructions (Bootzin, 1972; Bootzin, Epstein, & Wood, 1991) using mindfulness principles. Similar to cognitive behavior therapy for insomnia (CBT-I), sleep consolidation and sleep reconditioning are the core behavioral components in MBTI. This chapter describes the lessons and activities in MBTI that guide participants through the process of reprogramming the brain for sleep.

Session 3: Paying Attention to Sleepiness and Wakefulness

Session 3 has three major themes. First, MBTI instructors should reinforce the participant's meditation practice and introduce walking meditation as a means of expanding the practice to become aware of the body in motion. Second, instructors should provide information to guide participants on discerning the state of sleepiness from other states such as fatigue or depression. Finally, instructors should provide instructions

EXHIBIT 6.1

Session 3 Outline

Theme: Paying Attention to Sleepiness and Wakefulness

Objectives
1. Reinforce participants' meditation practice and introduce walking meditation.
2. Explain concepts of sleepiness, fatigue, and wakefulness.
3. Provide instructions for sleep consolidation.

Activities
1. Meditation Practice and Inquiry
   a. Walking meditation
   b. Body scan
   c. Inquiry and discussion of meditation practices

   Key Point: Introduce walking meditation as a means of mindful movement.

2. Insomnia Didactics and Strategies
   a. Provide instructions for sleep consolidation.

   Key Point: Make the connection between the awareness of sleepiness and using this awareness to follow sleep consolidation instructions.

Homework for Session 3
1. Complete sleep and meditation diaries.
2. Alternate walking meditation and body scan for at least 6 days (30 minutes per day).
3. Follow the sleep consolidation program.

for sleep consolidation as a strategy to begin reprogramming the brain for sleep. See Exhibit 6.1 for the Session 3 outline.

WALKING MEDITATION

Following the structure established in Session 2, the first hour of Session 3 is spent on the meditation practice. In Session 3, MBTI instructors should begin by introducing the walking meditation. The purpose of this meditation practice is to bring mindful awareness to the process of walking. When introducing the walking meditation, it might be helpful to first ask participants to describe how they normally walk. Most people will have difficulty describing details about walking because they do this automatically, without much thought or effort. In other words, the default mode is to walk mindlessly. This sets the stage for using the walking meditation as a practice to bring full awareness to the process of walking. See Exhibit 6.2 for instructions on leading the walking meditation.

During the period of inquiry following the first walking meditation, it is important to allow the participants to process their first experience

---

EXHIBIT 6.2

Walking Meditation

Notes: The walking meditation is introduced as a means of mindful movement, allowing participants to expand the repertoire of meditations and also to begin discovering mindfulness with the body in motion. To prepare for a walking meditation, instructors should first make sure that there is space for participants to walk around without bumping into objects or each other. If the situation allows, walking meditation can be done outside. If space is tight, it is sometimes possible to have participants walk around their mats or around a table. Also, instructors should engage in the walking meditation practice with the participants. The typical duration of this meditation is about 20 to 30 minutes.

Instructions:
1. Begin by having participants start in a mountain pose with feet about shoulder-width apart, hands straight down the sides, and the eyes looking straight ahead or slightly downward.
2. Have participants take a mindful breath and take a moment to notice any thoughts, feelings, and physical sensations that are present. This can be done with the eyes open or closed.
3. With eyes open, instruct participants to very slowly take one step forward, paying attention to sensations created with this first slow step.
4. Slowly, have participants take another step, then another, while bringing full awareness to the body in motion.
5. Have participants continue on their own, taking intentional slow steps. During the first walking meditation, instructors can provide periodic guidance on certain issues that often arise. For example, noticing what happens when we lose our balance while walking slowly or how the mind tends to jump to something other than walking. If these occur, just gently redirect the attention back to walking.
6. After a few minutes, participants can be encouraged to explore walking in different ways—backwards, sideways—or at a different pace.
7. End the walking meditation after about 20 to 30 minutes by ringing the bells.

Additional instructions and variations:
1. If weather permits, the walking meditation can be done outside.
2. Ask participants to pay close attention to their balance and note what happens when their mind has wandered.
3. Walking meditation is a reminder that we can generalize meditation exercises to various aspects of our daily lives without adding to the time constraints of our busy schedules.

---

with the walking meditation. Quite often comments will come up, such as "I don't think I have ever paid that much attention to walking" or "That was really annoying to walk so slowly." During this period of inquiry, instructors might ask the following questions:

- Did you notice anything different or new about the way you walk?
- Was it difficult to maintain balance? How is this different from the way you normally walk?
- How do you think walking this way might help you cope with insomnia?

Again, the purpose of the walking meditation and the discussion is to help participants recognize the contrast between their normal way of walking and practicing walking with mindful awareness.

Some participants prefer walking meditations over sitting meditations because they find it easier to maintain attention when there is something to focus on, such as movement. Others find the walking meditation difficult because they are not accustomed to walking so slowly or they find it difficult to maintain attention on a concept such as movement. If participants begin to express preferences regarding meditation types, gently encourage them to just follow the recommended practice without judging. Instructors should avoid trying to "push" participants toward one meditation or another but, instead, should allow participants to explore on their own what they can learn about themselves with each of the meditation practices. In the spirit of nonattachment, there is no preference for the type of meditation practice, but simply that one practices meditation.

After the period of inquiry for the walking meditation, a quiet meditation should follow. If time is short, instructors can lead a 15- to 20-minute sitting meditation. If more time is available, a full body scan meditation can be conducted. Starting from Session 3, the period of meditation usually involves one quiet and one movement practice. MBTI instructors can choose to manage the amount of time spent in each meditation and also the types of meditation. The recommended outline is provided as a suggestion in terms of what has worked well based on previous experience and other mindfulness-based programs. The didactic portion in Session 3 consists of discerning the state of sleepiness and providing instructions for sleep consolidation.

DISCERNING THE STATE OF SLEEPINESS

In MBTI, the discernment between sleepiness and fatigue (or other states of wakefulness) is vital for using mindfulness skills to work with insomnia. Recall from Chapter 1 that sleepiness represents a true physiological need for sleep. Therefore, it is an internal signal from the systems in the brain that provides important information about the brain's "readiness" for sleep to happen. This is a valuable cue if one pays attention to it. Bringing awareness to the presence or absence of sleepiness can provide guidance on managing sleep-related behaviors at that moment. For example, the presence of sleepiness is an indicator for going to bed, and the absence of sleepiness while in bed at night can be an indicator to get out of bed. This connection between the state of sleepiness and behaviors that regulate sleep is an important step toward reprogramming the brain for sleep.

How does meditation aid in recognizing the state of sleepiness? During mindfulness meditation practice, awareness can be directed to discern sensations associated with sleepiness from fatigue or other states of wakefulness. The principles of nonjudgmental awareness still apply—the goal is to not look for sleepiness. Nor are the sensations of sleepiness preferred over the sensations of fatigue. Instead, mindfulness practice allows one to examine what is present and to perceive the nature of those sensations with clarity. Discerning these sensations will allow for a more intentional response. The presence of sleepiness provides a greater chance of falling asleep at the beginning of the night or falling back to sleep in the middle of the night. In contrast, the presence of fatigue might indicate a need to rest or stop an activity, but it does not provide a greater chance of falling asleep. For many people with insomnia, the presence of either sleepiness or fatigue results in an automatic reaction of wanting to go to bed. As a result, the desire to escape wakefulness and the attachment to sleep becomes automatic and further perpetuates the symptoms of insomnia. This becomes a form of avoiding wakefulness that was discussed in Chapter 4. Therefore, awareness of these sensations becomes the first step in using mindful awareness to regulate sleep-related thoughts and behaviors.

Taking mindful action within the MBTI program involves the use of behavioral strategies for insomnia based on discerning the state of sleepiness. These strategies have been previously developed and tested as stand-alone treatments for insomnia and are also delivered as components of CBT-I. However, the use of mindful awareness in MBTI to recognize sleepiness is uniquely integrated into the behavioral strategies. Although both stimulus control and sleep restriction include instructions of not going to bed until sleepy, there is no explicit strategy or activity for teaching the patient how to identify the state of sleepiness. Anecdotally, some CBT-I therapists will provide information in a didactic manner to help patients understand the concept of sleepiness. Whereas a conceptual understanding of sleepiness can be useful for some people, others are not able to really understand the concept until there is an opportunity to have firsthand experience of sleepiness during treatment. In MBTI, the meditation practices are used as opportunities to experience firsthand the sensations of sleepiness as it arises so that the patient can better connect with their own experience of these sensations rather than just having a conceptual understanding of these sensations. The role of the MBTI instructor is to facilitate the connection between the conceptual understanding of sleepiness and the experience of sleepiness and other sensations. This experiential approach is consistent with a patient-centered framework by allowing patients to discover sleepiness in their own way.

SLEEP CONSOLIDATION

Sleep consolidation is a behavioral strategy for systematically adjusting the time spent in bed. It is adapted from the sleep restriction therapy developed by Spielman and colleagues (1987). Recall from Chapter 2 that sleep restriction therapy was based on the principle that people with insomnia tend to spend too much time in bed (TIB) as a reaction to difficulty sleeping. Unfortunately, the strategy of "casting a wider net to catch sleep" is actually disruptive to sleep physiology. Specifically, spending excessive TIB (usually more than 9 hours) reduces the homeostatic drive to sleep (Process S; see Chapter 1). With reduced homeostatic drive to sleep, sleep disturbance is actually more likely because there is less homeostatic pressure to maintain sleep during a prolonged period of TIB. As a result, casting a wider net actually perpetuates the problem of insomnia. In sleep restriction therapy, TIB is reduced to better match the amount of sleep time the individual is currently experiencing. Although this might initially lead to less total sleep time (TST), restricting TIB takes advantage of the homeostatic drive to sleep, such that the increased sleep drive serves to reduce the total wake time in bed. Gradually, TIB is systematically expanded as the patient experiences less total wake time.

Before providing specific instructions, MBTI instructors should convey three important points for following the sleep consolidation program. First, consistency with the instructions is vital. Much like making any change to a habit, a commitment to implementing the change can help promote adherence, even when the conditions are not desirable. This is especially true when the patient experiences a night of poor sleep and the desire to adjust the following night's bedtime or wake-up time is particularly tempting. Second, it is possible that participants will experience some daytime sleepiness or fatigue during this process. This is now recognized as a potential side effect of sleep restriction therapy (Kyle, Morgan, Spiegelhalder, & Espie, 2011). Therefore, MBTI instructors should caution participants to be aware of this possibility and to take appropriate action to avoid operating motor vehicles or other potential consequences of daytime sleepiness. The third point is to ease concerns that the initial sleep window is not a permanent schedule but a starting point. Some patients get very anxious that this will be their permanent sleep schedule. Instructors can reduce these fears by explaining that sleep consolidation is a dynamic process and the schedule will be revisited weekly and adjustments made as their sleep patterns begin to change.

In MBTI, sleep restriction instructions have been modified to align with the principles of mindfulness (see Exhibit 6.3 for a summary of these instructions). Establishing the importance of a regular and consistent rise

Instructions for Sleep Consolidation Program

Notes: It is important to help each participant choose a rise time and a bedtime that are reasonable and have a good chance to succeed. In doing so, have the participant consider both ends of the window. He or she may initially decide that 7:00 a.m. is a desirable wake-up time. However, if the initial time in bed (TIB) prescription is 6 hours, this rise time would result in an earliest bedtime of 1:00 a.m. Upon discovering this fact, the participant may wish to select an earlier wake-up time so that bedtime can be earlier during the night. The instructor might want to do this during the large group discussion or go around the room and help each dyad. Also note that compliance with the TIB prescription will usually be best when the participant takes an active role in selecting the sleep window. The instructions below can be used with Handout 5 in the Appendix.

Instructions:
1. Begin with establishing a regular rise time (or wake-up time). Emphasize that this is a fixed time, regardless of the amount of sleep or how one feels upon waking up. It is best to choose a wake-up time that is reasonable for the individual and fits his or her lifestyle. Once a wake-up time is selected, it will be maintained for the next week, including weekends or off days. Instructors can refer to Handout 5 as a guide to help explain the instructions and answer questions about establishing a regular wake-up time.
2. Determine the sleep window, which will be the amount of time allowed to spend in bed. To determine the initial TIB window, the average total sleep time (TST) reported by the patient on his/her current sleep diary is calculated. Subsequently, the initial TIB window is determined using the formula: TIB = average TST + 30 minutes. Adding 30 minutes to the average TST allows for normal sleep onset latency and brief nocturnal arousals. Handout 5 also shows the formula to determine the sleep window.
3. Once the sleep window is determined, remind participants that TIB is anchored by the rise time in the morning and a recommended bedtime at night. If this timing does not seem reasonable to the participant, discuss possible adjustments. Keeping a tighter window (i.e., shorter TIB) is usually preferred because it provides the best opportunity to decrease wakefulness.
4. Review sleep consolidation instructions if necessary and see if there are any questions. Then break into pairs or small groups to allow participants to discuss setting their own sleep window. Come back and discuss each person's sleep consolidation schedule.

time (i.e., time getting out of bed to start the day) is the first step. This rise time does not need to be earlier than the current wake-up time, but the consistency of getting out of bed at this time is emphasized. Sometimes "negotiations" will happen, as it is important to strike a balance between a rise time that is more consistent with the participant's circadian rhythm and one that can be feasibly sustained on a regular basis. My approach is to select a schedule that balances the likelihood of initial success with one that is realistic given the patient's level of motivation and lifestyle factors. Once a consistent rise time has been established, then a *sleep window* is discussed as the period for time in bed (TIB). The instructions for calculating this sleep window are typically based on TST averaged across the most recent week (or 2 weeks) reported in the patient's sleep diaries. Thirty minutes are then added to the average TST, to come up with the recommended TIB. For example, if the average TST on the sleep diary is 5 hours, then the TIB would be 5.5 hours, or 330 minutes in bed. Once the window is established, it is crucial to emphasize that the beginning of the sleep window is not a set time to go to bed. It is very important to pay attention to the state of sleepiness at this time. If the sensations of sleepiness are present such that there is a high probability of falling asleep, then it is appropriate to go to bed. However, if the beginning of the sleep window arrives and sleepiness is not yet present, then bedtime should be delayed until these sensations emerge. It is possible to engage in a meditation practice around this time to help bring awareness to the mental and physical states. The key is to become aware of the internal cues that determine when to go to bed, rather than external cues, such as the clock, that are not directly related to the probability of falling asleep. It is important to note that if sleepiness emerges before the sleep window, bedtime should still be delayed until the beginning of the sleep window. This principle is important to establish regularity of the window.

After the instructions for sleep consolidation are explained, some further negotiations might be necessary. For example, the placement of the sleep window might need to be adjusted to account for lifestyle preferences, work schedules, or school schedules. It is also important to emphasize that the initial goal of sleep consolidation is to decrease total wake time rather than to increase TST. For safety reasons, TIB is usually not reduced to less than 5 hours. Even if participants have an average TST below 5 hours, limiting TIB below 5 hours might lead to excessive daytime sleepiness that could put the participant at risk for accidents or adverse events related to sleepiness. Therefore, caution is warranted for these participants by keeping the minimum TIB at 5 hours. Finally, the importance of consistency during this time should be reinforced. Analogous to training a new pet, the brain needs to have consistent reinforcement to adjust to this new sleep phase. Ultimately, the sleep consolidation program will provide patients with a method for determining their own sleep needs.

In MBTI, instructors should first provide the rationale and instructions for sleep consolidation and then allow participants to choose their own schedule using Handout 5 (see the Appendix). Normally, participants discuss their schedule in pairs and then report back to the group. The instructor can provide guidance when the patient has not applied the instructions correctly or if the schedule is clearly not helpful. Instructors should encourage participants to manage their own sleep consolidation program for several reasons: (a) doing so establishes an opportunity to further discover sleep in a manner consistent with the mindfulness principles; (b) patients are more likely to adhere to their own schedule if it is set by themselves rather than prescribed by the instructor; (c) setting their own schedules can enhance patient engagement and self-efficacy. Finally, it is important to remind participants to keep recording their sleep and bedtime patterns in the sleep diaries. Review of progress depends on the data from the sleep diaries. When participants do not bring in complete sleep diaries, then the sleep consolidation program is not as precise and might not be as effective.

HOMEWORK FOR SESSION 3

The recommended homework assignment for Session 3 is to alternate the walking meditation and body scan meditation for at least 30 minutes per day, 6 days out of the week. This allows participants to have some variety in their meditation practice. In addition, participants are asked to follow the sleep window they developed as part of the sleep consolidation program. Finally, participants should continue to keep recording in their sleep and meditation diaries.

Session 4: Working With Sleeplessness at Night

The first theme for Session 4 is to teach participants mindful movement through stretching and light yoga. The second theme is to review the initial sleep schedules from the sleep consolidation instructions and to discuss how to make adjustments on the basis of the sleep diary data. The third theme is to introduce sleep reconditioning as a behavioral strategy for working with sleeplessness at night. See Exhibit 6.4 for an outline of Session 4.

YOGA OR MINDFUL STRETCHING

The movement meditation for Session 4 involves either light yoga or gentle stretching. The choice of which meditation practice to lead depends on the instructor's background and comfort with these practices. Much like mindfulness-based stress reduction (MBSR), the practice of yoga in MBTI is not meant to replace or teach formal yoga practices. The purpose is to bring mindful awareness to the body as it moves and stretches in different poses. Since many participants will not have had experience with yoga, it might be helpful to explain that the intention in MBTI is not to teach formal yoga practices, but that some of the poses used in MBTI are borrowed from hatha yoga.

Session 4 Outline

Theme: Working With Sleeplessness at Night

Objectives
1. Provide instructions for mindful movement.
2. Review sleep consolidation and provide instructions for adjusting the sleep window.
3. Provide instructions for using sleep reconditioning to work with sleeplessness.

Activities
1. Meditation Practice and Inquiry
   a. Introduce mindful movement and stretching (light yoga)
   b. Sitting meditation
   c. Inquiry and discussion of meditation practices

   Key Point: Introduce yoga/light stretching as a mindful movement practice.

2. Insomnia Didactics and Strategies
   a. Review progress with initial sleep consolidation and make adjustments as needed.
   b. Provide instructions for sleep reconditioning.

   Key Point: Provide rationale and instructions for sleep reconditioning. Emphasize the connections with the ongoing practice of awareness of sleepiness and wakefulness.

Homework for Session 4
1. Complete sleep and meditation diaries.
2. Alternate mindful movement and sitting meditation for at least 6 days (30 minutes per day).
3. Follow sleep consolidation and sleep reconditioning instructions.

The gentle stretching is a series of stretches that I developed on the bases of my own movement meditation practice and my experience as a personal trainer. The purpose is similar to that of hatha yoga, except that these are simple stretches that might be less intimidating for an instructor without experience teaching yoga. I do incorporate a few yoga poses (e.g., mountain pose, child's pose, table pose) into the sequence, but I do not have any formal training in yoga myself. The set of stretches that I have used in MBTI is listed in Exhibit 6.5.

Instructors should pay attention to a few issues when leading yoga or mindful stretching. First, it is important to guide the class slowly through a sequence of postures or stretches, with appropriate teaching comments interspersed as needed. Verbal guidance should be explicit and accurate so that participants know what to do without having to look at the instructor all the time. The instructor might first need to practice alone or lead a mindful movement session with family or friends before leading a class. Second, it is important to encourage participants to be conservative and to listen carefully to their own bodies. Emphasis is placed on mindfulness and approaching one's limits with

EXHIBIT 6.5

Mindful Movement Exercises

Notes: Before starting the mindful movement exercises, remind participants to keep in mind the principles of mindfulness. This includes approaching this as a "non–goal-oriented exercise" by keeping a perspective of acceptance, non-striving, and beginner's mind. Also, remind participants to pay attention to their bodies and work within their limitations. Note the limitations, and do not push beyond the body's capabilities at this time. On the other hand, encourage participants to gently explore their limits and the body's capabilities right now, not what it used to be. Be aware of instances where pain or injury to the body in the past has led to protecting ourselves by backing off or restricting movement.

Sample exercises for mindful stretching and moving:

While standing
1. Mountain pose
2. Neck rolls
3. Shoulder rolls
4. Arm circles
5. Stretching upward and slowly let the arms down to the side
6. Gentle twist from side to side
7. Squats or deep knee bends

While on hands and knees on the mat
1. Cow pose (inhale, head looks up, curve in the lower back, toes curl in)
2. Cat pose (exhale, head looks in, toes point out, round back)
3. Stretch shoulders and back

While lying on the mat
1. Corpse pose (palms facing up, stretching body out)
2. Stretching—hamstring, (each leg), hip flexors (each leg), arms outstretched (back and shoulders)
3. Bridge—arching the back and doing the bridge

---

gentleness. Therefore, participants should avoid any postures they feel would cause injury or a setback, and they should be instructed to experiment very cautiously when in doubt. Instructors should pay particular attention to people with lower back or neck problems and to people with general chronic pain. Finally, it is important to maintain the principle of nonjudgmental awareness. Participants might comment that they are not doing a pose or stretch correctly by saying, "I can't seem to do this pose" or "I am not flexible enough to do this stretch." If such comments are made, instructors can remind participants that there is no right or wrong way to meditate. As long as participants are bringing mindful awareness to their body's movement and limits, then they are practicing mindfulness meditation.

By the end of Session 4, all formal meditations should have been introduced and led at least once during the session so that participants have had the opportunity to experience the complete set of guided meditations for MBTI. Moving forward, the first hour of MBTI consists of two meditation practices, typically one quiet meditation and one movement meditation. MBTI instructors can select which meditations seem most appropriate given the dynamics of the class. Instructors might also vary the setting, doing a walking meditation outside or in the hallway (if appropriate) or even conduct sitting meditations in chairs rather than on the ground. These are done in the spirit of beginner's mind, so that each meditation practice is seen as a new practice, even if the type of meditation has been practiced many times by participants throughout MBTI. During the period of inquiry, it is important that the instructor continues to practice mindful listening. It is tempting to use certain comments from participants as teaching points, but this is not the purpose of the period of inquiry. Instead, the instructor can point out interesting insights that the participants report, but she or he should refrain from expressing preferences regarding the participants' experiences (e.g., who is doing it right or wrong).

REVIEWING AND ADJUSTING THE SLEEP CONSOLIDATION WINDOW

The insomnia-related didactic portion of Session 4 should start with a review of the sleep consolidation schedule that was assigned in Session 3. This review will continue in Sessions 5, 6, and 7, so it is important to set a precedent for how to review the schedule and make changes. The sleep consolidation program is reviewed on a weekly basis using the participant's sleep diaries to discuss progress and the need to make adjustments to the sleep window. It is very important to review progress and reinforce the concepts of sleep consolidation when they return after the first week of following the sleep window. This allows the instructor to examine how consistently participants have adhered to the sleep window. First, consistency of the rise time is important to monitor. Because many people with insomnia are used to sleeping in whenever they can during weekends or days off work, consistency on these days is especially important for the instructor to review. If participants are hesitant about getting out of bed or complain that they are not likely to "make up for lost sleep," it is important to remind them that the inconsistency is likely to confuse the brain. Much like training a pet, consistency is important for the brain to understand that we are trying to establish a fixed rise time. Delaying the wake-up time by more than an hour can create the effect of social jet lag that was described in Chapter 1. The result is an inconsistent rhythm that mimics travel across several time zones during the weekend or off days.

A second common mistake is that participants think that the beginning of the sleep window is the time they should be going to bed, and hence they continue to experience prolonged sleep onset latency after they go to bed. This is usually detectable by reviewing the sleep diaries. If bedtime is the same time, or nearly the same time, as the beginning of the sleep window, and sleep onset is prolonged (e.g., for more than 30 minutes), then it is helpful to ask participants how they decided when to go to bed. Most often they will report following the sleep consolidation schedule. If this is the case, then it is important to review the instructions, emphasizing that while the morning rise time is fixed and should be followed consistently, the beginning of the window represents the earliest time that one can go to bed. The key to determining when to go to bed is based on an awareness of the mental and physical states at that time. If sleepiness is not yet present, it is better to delay bedtime until it is. If the sensation of sleepiness is present at the beginning of the sleep window, then it serves as a signal from the body that it is ready for sleep. MBTI instructors should reinforce the connection between identification of sleepiness and the behavioral strategies as needed.

A third common mistake is that participants keep the duration of the sleep window intact but decide to move the position of the sleep window from day to day. For example, the sleep diary might show that the individual is spending only 6 hours in bed, as agreed on for the sleep window. However, review of the diaries indicates that on Monday night the 6 hours occurred between 12:00 a.m. and 6:00 a.m.; on Tuesday night the 6 hours occurred between 1:00 a.m. and 7:00 a.m.; and on the weekends the 6 hours occurred between 3:00 a.m. and 9:00 a.m. It is important to reinforce the importance of keeping the timing or position of the window steady. If it moves several hours, it could still create social jet lag. Also, moving the sleep window frequently tends to be a reaction caused by poor sleep, social activities, trying even harder to control sleep, or a misunderstanding of the purpose of the sleep consolidation program. Here, it might be helpful to explain that following the sleep consolidation window at the same time removes the "thinking" behind deciding how to compensate for poor sleep and instead, remaining steady with the sleep window actually helps to cultivate self-efficacy regarding sleep. Rather than continuing to chase sleep or reacting to sleep disturbance, the sleep consolidation schedule is designed to provide the optimal conditions for sleep to occur during a prespecified window. Over time, this allows the brain to become reprogrammed for sleep.

The concept of sleep efficiency is usually introduced in Session 4 during the review of the initial sleep consolidation schedule. Sleep efficiency is explained to participants as a way to calculate how efficiently

we are spending our time in bed. The formula for sleep efficiency (SE)
is $SE = \dfrac{TST}{TIB} \times 100$

As can be seen from the formula, sleep efficiency is a percentage
of actual sleep time during the time spent in bed. Optimizing sleep efficiency is one of the goals of the sleep consolidation program. Often participants are anxious or skeptical, believing that spending less time in
bed results in decreased TST, thus their sleep efficiencies remain low.
However, sleep research indicates that spending less time in bed increases
the homeostatic pressure for sleep, thus increasing the likelihood of
sleeping (Spielman et al., 1987). Although there might be an occasional
night during which TST is indeed low, it is highly unlikely that this trend
would continue over several nights. Furthermore, sleep efficiency is an
index that is partly controllable (TIB), whereas attachment to total sleep
time is likely to remain unpredictable and uncontrollable. In this way,
the sleep consolidation program can promote a shift in sleep-related
metacognition.

After explaining the concept of sleep efficiency, the instructor should
demonstrate how this can be calculated from the sleep diaries. It is helpful to bring calculators to this session. Participants are instructed to calculate their sleep efficiency for each night of the last week and then take
the average to calculate the sleep efficiency for the entire week. This
average sleep efficiency is then used to determine whether changes to
the sleep window are needed. (The instructions for adjusting the sleep
window are provided in the Appendix, Handout 6.) In general, the interpretation of sleep efficiencies fall into categories that are similar to the
*A*s, *B*s, and *C*s on school exams. Changes to the sleep window are normally made in small increments, either 15 minutes or 30 minutes, at most.
The sleep window is increased for participants who report sleep efficiencies in the "*A* range" (sleep efficiency 90% or higher), accompanied by
a self-report of feeling sleepy during the day. Together, these are indica-
tors that the participant's sleep drive is high and they are likely getting
insufficient sleep. The instructor then discusses whether the additional
time should be added at the beginning of the sleep window or at its end.
Determination for where to add the additional time depends on several
factors, including lifestyle preferences, work schedules, considerations
for children's or a partner's schedules, as well as a person's *chronotype* (i.e.,
his or her preference for morning or evening activities). Frequently, the
decision is made on the basis of practical considerations. For example, a
working adult who must get out of bed by 6:00 a.m. each weekday morning will need to add the 15 minutes by advancing the bedtime 15 minutes
earlier. Determination for the amount of time to add depends on the
degree of sleepiness and clinician judgment as to the likely benefit of an
increased window. One rule of thumb to follow is that the tighter the

sleep window, the faster the results usually happen. Spending less time in bed allows the sleep drive (Process S) to accumulate over a longer period of wakefulness, resulting in a more potent appetite for sleep. In essence, this is a controlled form of partial sleep deprivation, which increases the probability that the sleep system will generate a high sleep efficiency during the sleep window. However, it is also more difficult to remain consistent in following a tighter sleep window. The wider the sleep window, the easier it is to follow, but the results might not happen as quickly. Clinicians should use these considerations to discuss with participants and come to a mutual agreement. Gaining the participant's perspective and participation in making the decision together will increase the likelihood that the participant will adhere to the schedule.

If the participant has a sleep efficiency in the "C range" (sleep efficiency less than 80%), the sleep window is normally reduced by 15 or 30 minutes. Sleep efficiencies in this range reflect that the window is still too wide and sleep is not sufficiently consolidated. If participants are reluctant to reduce TIB, it might be helpful to remind them that this is a temporary tool and that once sleep efficiencies increase, TIB can be increased. Recall that the minimum TIB is usually 5 hours because of safety concerns related to excessive daytime sleepiness. Even if participants have low sleep efficiencies with this amount of time in bed, it might be prudent to allow them to remain at the same sleep schedule for another week. Another option for these participants is to combine sleep consolidation with sleep reconditioning (which is described subsequently).

If the participant has a sleep efficiency in the "B range" (less than 90% and 80% or higher), the sleep window is usually kept constant for another week. The rationale is that it might be best to stay at this window for another week to collect more data and see if sleep efficiencies will improve. Some patients might choose to be more aggressive and are willing to reduce TIB in an effort to improve sleep efficiency more quickly. This is permissible, but the decision should be made with the patient's approval to enhance motivation. Instructors can use discretion as to whether or not the patient is ready to make adjustments.

After they receive instructions for how to make changes to their sleep window, participants are encouraged to discuss in pairs or small groups how they wish to implement these changes during the next week. After 5 to 10 minutes of discussion with their partner, each participant reports to the group what adjustments they would like to make to their schedule for the next week. The instructor should provide guidance when questions arise and assess for safety concerns (e.g., excessive daytime sleepiness, symptoms of mania or depression). As with the period of inquiry, the MBTI instructor should listen mindfully as each participant provides an update and should not interfere unnecessarily with the participant's selected schedule.

The sleep consolidation program can be a powerful behavioral strategy within MBTI. Yet, it can also facilitate metacognitive shifts in several ways. First, directing attention to sleep efficiency rather than TST provides a shift in the conceptualization of sleep needs. By shifting thoughts away from TST—a sleep parameter that is not directly controllable—and toward sleep efficiency, a sleep parameter in which TIB can be controlled, participants learn to bring attention to how they are using their TIB rather than to how much they are sleeping. For example, sleep efficiency can be increased by reducing TIB, even if TST remains the same. It also reinforces the principles of nonattachment to sleep, as now there is a window set aside and one simply allows for sleep to "fill up that window." Although sleep might not completely fill up that window every night, establishing a regular window provides a greater probability of sleep occurring during this period. Finally, sleep consolidation reinforces the notion of beginner's mind by shifting the approach from trying to achieve a certain amount of sleep to discovering one's sleep needs within a scheduled window. The process of adjusting the sleep window serves as a self-directed experiment to determine one's own sleep timing and sleep needs. Rather than relying on the media or scientific reports that advise on the average amount of sleep needed, this provides a systematic method of determining one's personal sleep needs. Much like trying on different shoes, it is about finding the shoe size that fits best for each person rather than finding the shoe that fits the average person. These explanations can also serve as ways to create metacognitive shifts and reduce secondary arousal in the context of insomnia.

SLEEP RECONDITIONING

The third major theme of Session 4 is to introduce the instructions for sleep reconditioning. Many people have heard that it is best to get out of bed if they cannot sleep. Some might have tried it on a few nights but found that it was not helpful. Others worry that it will make their sleep problem worse. Most people do not understand the theory and rationale behind these instructions, which come from a behavioral intervention known as *stimulus control* (Bootzin, 1972; Bootzin, Epstein, & Wood, 1991). This intervention was first introduced in Chapter 2 and is based on the theory of conditioned arousal. In the context of normal sleep, the bed and bedroom serve as cues, or stimuli, that are associated with relaxation, sleepiness, and security, which promote sleep. However, as insomnia develops and the experience of difficulty falling asleep at the beginning of the night or falling back to sleep in the middle of the night becomes more frequent, frustration and anxiety emerge while the person is lying in bed trying to sleep. Over time, the feelings of frustration and anxiety become associated with the bedroom environment, and this environment is no longer a discriminative stimulus for sleep. This association creates conditioned performance anxiety in which the condition (bedroom) to perform (go to sleep) creates anxiety and difficulty, further preventing effective performance (sleeping). As a way to extinguish the conditioned performance anxiety and reestablish the bed and bedroom as discriminative stimuli for sleep, the original instructions for stimulus control involve getting out of bed when unable to sleep and returning to bed only when sleepy. As an extension, the bed is not used for anything except for sleep. For example, eating, working, and watching TV in bed are prohibited. The one exception to the rule is sexual activity. Finally, the wake-up time should be fixed, regardless of the amount of sleep obtained during the night. Over time, the stimulus control instructions are designed to decrease the conditioned arousal and reestablish the discriminative value of the bed and bedroom to promote sleep.

In MBTI, sleep reconditioning adapts the essential instructions of stimulus control with a delivery that fits the framework of mindfulness principles. Instructions for sleep reconditioning are provided in the Appendix (Handout 7), which should be given to participants. Similar to providing instructions for sleep consolidation, it is paramount for MBTI instructors to emphasize the importance of recognizing the state of sleepiness when following the instructions for sleep reconditioning. Without understanding the sensations associated with sleepiness, the sleep reconditioning instructions would not be effective because of the theory behind reconditioning the bedroom environment with sleepiness. In MBTI, the meditations serve as a means of cultivating greater awareness of the state of sleepiness and being able to discern it from other states, such as fatigue or depression. Once again, awareness becomes the platform for deciding how to engage in sleep-related behaviors. In this case, awareness of sleepiness helps to determine whether one is ready to go to bed, which is based on the presence or absence of sleepiness at that moment. If sleepiness is not present when lying in bed, then the probability of falling asleep is low, and it would be important to get out of sleep mode (see the Appendix, Handout 7, Step 2). Ideally, it would be best to leave the bed and bedroom. Once out of sleep mode, one should engage in a soothing, relaxing activity for the sake of enjoying the activity, not for the sake of enabling a return to bed. Staying in dim light can also avoid disturbances to the circadian system (Process C). It can be difficult to find an activity to do in the middle of the night without wanting to go back to bed. Some activities that patients have found to be helpful include knitting, crochet, or reading something light (e.g., magazine, comic book). One common mistake in implementing these instructions is to use a boring activity, as opposed to a soothing activity, and to simply count the minutes (or hours) before one can return to bed. A patient once told me that he would get out of bed to read the telephone book in the middle of the night. When I asked him if he found this to be soothing, he said, "No! I hated myself for having to read the phone book to fall asleep!" Clearly, this patient's approach is inconsistent with mindfulness and is not likely to be helpful, as it does not remove the effort to sleep and is not grounded in self-compassion. Therefore, it is important to have a discussion with participants regarding what to do when they choose to get out of bed. The third step (see the Appendix, Handout 7, Step 3) is to return to bed when sleepy. Again, awareness of the sensations of sleepiness rather than the clock time should be used to decide when to return to bed. Many people will worry that if they do not go back to bed within 30 minutes or a certain amount of time, then they will remain awake the rest of the night. This possibility should be acknowledged, but it is unlikely to persist night after night because of the homeostatic drive for sleep. Finally, it is important to reinforce the instructions of avoiding waking activities while in bed. This includes watching television, using a portable electronic device (e.g., laptop, tablet, cell phone), eating, studying, or doing work.

MBTI instructors should be cognizant of a few important issues related to delivering sleep reconditioning instructions. First, the importance of following these instructions consistently should be emphasized. Furthermore, it should be emphasized that these instructions can be used more than one time per night. Much like sleep consolidation, inconsistent application of this technique is not likely to yield consistent changes in sleep. In some cases, it might be better to allow participants the option of choosing to follow the sleep reconditioning instructions or the sleep consolidation window. A guiding principle for making this decision is that the sleep window is an a priori decision, such that the window is set for the entire week. This might be more helpful for participants who are still experiencing persistent sleep difficulties on a nightly basis. Sleep reconditioning instructions can be implemented on a conditional basis, if sleep problems occur on any given night. Thus, participants who have a more variable pattern of sleep disruption might prefer to follow sleep reconditioning instructions, as they only have to implement them on the nights were sleep disruption is significant. For example, a participant who experiences prolonged awakenings in the middle of the night three nights out of the week, but not on the other nights, would only have to use sleep reconditioning on those three nights.

A second consideration is to discuss what activities are permissible when getting out of bed. The question of reading and watching television is a very common one. In the spirit of mindfulness, I normally suggest that the activities can vary between individuals, but the important principle is to find something soothing and pleasant and not something that promotes sleep effort. Frequently, this leads to the question of practicing meditation as an activity for sleep reconditioning. This can be a difficult choice and might depend on the progress the participant has made in his or her own meditation practice. If the participant appears to understand the principles and seems to be able to apply the principles of mindfulness during meditations at night, then it would be fine to allow meditation practice as part of sleep reconditioning. However, if the participant seems to be using the meditation as a way to help go back to sleep, then the principle of nonattachment to sleep would be violated, and it would be best not to practice meditation during these nocturnal awakenings.

Finally, the question of whether or not one has to get out of bed should be addressed. An experiment conducted many years ago provided insight into this question. Zwart and Lisman (1979) conducted a study of 47 undergraduates assigned to stimulus control (all instructions), temporal control (lie down only when sleepy, rise at the same time each day, do not nap), noncontingent control (a fixed number of risings from bed within 20 minutes of going to bed), countercontrol (sit up in bed and read, watch TV, etc., if unable to sleep), or no treatment. They found countercontrol as effective as stimulus control, suggesting that doing a different activity when unable to sleep is sufficient to eliminate the association of the bed as a cue for arousal. Therefore, it seems that the important "ingredient" of sleep reconditioning is to "get out of sleep mode" rather than getting out of the bed.

Similar to the activity for sleep consolidation, it can be useful to have participants break into pairs or small groups to discuss how they wish to implement the sleep reconditioning program. Participants should be encouraged to discuss what they will do when they get out of bed or when they will choose to get out of bed. Instructors should provide guidance without specifically telling the participants what to do. Again, this follows a patient-centered approach to facilitate mindful discovery of how these strategies can be implemented in their individual situations.

HOMEWORK FOR SESSION 4

The homework assignment for Session 4 is to alternate mindful movement with sitting meditation for 30 minutes a day, at least 6 days out of the week. In addition, participants are asked to follow the changes to their sleep consolidation program and to follow the instructions for sleep reconditioning. Finally, participants are asked to continue with the sleep and meditation diaries. Participants should begin to see how these diaries are used in the MBTI program to inform the behavioral components.

By the end of Session 4, participants will have experienced at least two quiet meditations and two movement meditations, which serve as the practice for cultivating awareness. They will also have the instructions for the two main behavioral components of sleep consolidation and sleep reconditioning, which provides a means of taking mindful action based on the awareness of the state of sleepiness. Although the concept of metacognitions might be discussed during some of the behavioral instructions, the focus of Sessions 5, 6, and 7 turns more directly to addressing metacognitions in the context of insomnia.

Using Mindfulness Principles to Work With the Territory of Insomnia

7

M indfulness-based therapy for insomnia (MBTI) often uses the term *shift* to refer to a subtle or small magnitude of change. This idea fits the metacognitive model of insomnia that was described in Chapter 4 and is an important feature of working with sleep-related arousal in MBTI. Expanding awareness to include metacognitions and then making incremental shifts in metacognitions can open up opportunities to see the problem of insomnia from different perspectives. In Session 5, the *territory of insomnia* is introduced to participants as a different way to think about the various domains (behavioral, cognitive, metacognitive) that are encompassed in the course of chronic insomnia. Sessions 6 and 7 explore other domains within the territory of insomnia, including acceptance and letting go, revising the relationship with sleep, and finding other ways to engage in self-compassion and self-care that do not directly involve getting more sleep. During these sessions, the focus is on applying mindfulness principles and practices to create metacognitive shifts in working with thoughts and feelings related to insomnia. Participants

http://dx.doi.org/10.1037/14952-008
Mindfulness-Based Therapy for Insomnia, by J. C. Ong

closely examine the way they approach both sleeping and waking stress, and when possible, find ways to shift out of a reactive mode that brings mindfulness into their daily lives. Furthermore, identification of personal values and examining choices that can be congruent with these values are discussed as a means of handling relapse prevention and potential future episodes of insomnia. Therefore, these sessions are grouped together in this chapter because they are aimed at metacognitive shifts using the mindfulness skills and practices that have been taught during the first half of MBTI.

Session 5: The Territory of Insomnia

THE HALFWAY POINT

Session 5 marks the halfway point in the MBTI program. By this time, participants should have a formal meditation practice established, and they should be familiar with the series of quiet and movement meditations that are used in MBTI. They should also be familiar with the behavioral strategies and be implementing sleep consolidation and sleep reconditioning at home.

Session 5 has three major themes. First, the halfway point offers an opportunity to reinforce the meditation practice and to encourage participants to recommit to the practice of meditation for the second half of the program. Second, continued discussions should occur about how to adjust the sleep consolidation and sleep reconditioning programs during the insomnia-related didactic portion of the session. The third theme is to introduce the concept of the territory of insomnia. The territory of insomnia serves as a model for making metacognitive shifts, such that participants are encouraged to use the platform of awareness to view the problem of insomnia in ways that might be different than before and to apply mindfulness principles to work with their own territory of insomnia. See Exhibit 7.1 for the Session 5 outline.

MEDITATION PRACTICE AND PERIOD OF INQUIRY

The meditation practice follows the structure for a movement meditation and a quiet meditation that was established during the first half of MBTI. Instructors might begin to experiment with subtle shifts in leading the meditation practice. For example, instructors might provide less guidance during a sitting meditation and encourage participants to explore whatever arises in the mind and body on their own. This is sometimes

---

EXHIBIT 7.1

Session 5 Outline

Theme: The Territory of Insomnia

Objectives
1. Encourage participants to make a recommitment to the meditation practice.
2. Discuss how to make adjustments to sleep consolidation and sleep reconditioning.
3. Explain the concept of the territory of insomnia.

Activities
1. Meditation Practice and Inquiry
     a. Movement meditation (walking meditation or mindful movement and stretching)
     b. Quiet meditation (body scan or sitting meditation)
     c. Inquiry and discussion of meditation practices
     d. Review of meditation practice at halfway point

   Key Point: Encourage participants to deepen their meditation practice.

2. Insomnia Didactics and Strategies
     a. Introduce and discuss the concept of the territory of insomnia.
     b. Review progress with sleep consolidation and make alterations as needed.
     c. Review progress with sleep reconditioning and reinforce instructions as needed.

   Key Point: Encourage participants to recognize that insomnia is more than just a problem of not sleeping at night.

Homework for Session 5
1. Complete sleep and meditation diaries.
2. Alternate between a movement meditation (mindful walking, yoga) and quiet meditation (sitting meditation, body scan) for at least 6 days (30 minutes per day).
3. Continue with sleep consolidation and sleep reconditioning instructions.

---

called a *choiceless awareness* meditation in which there is more silence and space for participants to provide self-guidance during the meditation practice. This is one way to "take off the training wheels" during the meditation practice and allow participants to practice self-guided meditations. Ultimately, participants should be able to conduct self-guided meditations rather than relying on guidance from an instructor or digital media for every meditation practice.

During the period of inquiry in Session 5, instructors should spend time checking in with participants to determine whether they are willing to recommit to continuing the meditation practice for the next 4 weeks. As they make this recommitment, participants can be reminded to let go of expectations for the second half of the program on the basis of the first half of the course. It is also an opportunity to practice beginner's mind. Instructors can facilitate a discussion on what participants have learned thus far in MBTI or if they have noticed any changes since starting MBTI. As participants have been practicing meditation for a few weeks at this point, many might begin to describe new discoveries of their mental and physical states. Below are quotes from past participants in MBTI groups. One participant commented at the halfway point:

> For several months, I would dread going to bed because I just didn't know how it [sleep] would go. During the last 2 weeks, I don't think I have had that same feeling of anticipation [of not sleeping].

Others might report that they are noticing more variability in their sensations of sleepiness and fatigue across the day. An example of this is described in the following paragraph.

> I used to feel sleepy and tired all the time, but I have noticed that it is not as constant as it used to be. I now feel more sleepy in the afternoon, but then feel more energetic later in the evening. Not sure if things have actually changed or if I am just seeing it differently.

Still others might comment on how they have noticed a tendency to automatically respond in a particular way. One participant made the following observation:

> After we learned about being on automatic pilot, I realized how reactive I am. I am still learning how to work with this but at least now I can see it. The breathing [meditation] is like a GPS for me.

Some participants might not report any new discoveries. In the spirit of practicing the mindfulness principle of nonjudging, instructors should acknowledge that it is fine not to have any new discoveries. This avoids inadvertently communicating to participants that having new discoveries is desirable, which could be perceived as a value judgement. The key is to encourage participants to continue with their meditation practice and just watch and see what arises. As these observations indicate, participants will often learn something about themselves or gain a different perspective about their symptoms of insomnia. Metacognitive awareness is the starting point for making metacognitive shifts.

INSOMNIA DIDACTICS AND TROUBLESHOOTING

During the insomnia didactic portion of Session 5, adjustments to the sleep consolidation and sleep reconditioning programs should continue as discussed in Chapter 6. Some participants might voice difficulties in adhering to the instructions. For example, a participant from one group stated that the thought of getting out of bed in the middle of the night was "repugnant," and he refused to do so. Others might have difficulty keeping a consistent wake-up time. The troubleshooting for these challenges can be done in small groups or pairs, followed by a group discussion. This allows participants to discuss their challenges with their peers and work together toward finding solutions. During the trouble-shooting process, MBTI instructors should practice mindfulness principles and reinforce the rationale of the instructions when needed but otherwise allow participants to discover solutions on their own. Exceptions should be made if a participant is not implementing the instructions correctly or if the instructor feels that there might be a potential risk to the participant. For example, a participant who sets a sleep window for only 4 hours might be at risk for excessive daytime sleepiness. Managing group discussions takes mindful practice to avoid wanting to immediately fix a sleep window that is not working for a participant. Often at least one group member will have seen improvements in his or her symptoms, and this person can then be very helpful in providing peer support and helping others problem solve. This scenario should be allowed to unfold organically; the MBTI instructor should not encourage one group member to help others.

THE TERRITORY OF INSOMNIA

Recall from Chapter 4 that the *territory of insomnia* refers to the entire range of symptoms, behaviors, thoughts, and values that encompass the experience of chronic insomnia. I selected this term intentionally because the word *territory* is not commonly used to describe a health condition, much less a sleep disorder. It stands out as being awkward or unusual, and people will ask, "What do you mean by the territory of insomnia?" Addressing this question provides an opportunity to reconsider the experience of insomnia from a mindful stance that is not bound by the criteria for insomnia disorders or the etiological models of chronic insomnia. This can involve a metacognitive shift and a practice of beginner's mind with regard to what insomnia means. Rather than just trying to sleep more or sleep better, seeing the entire territory of insomnia allows participants the opportunity to more effectively use the skills they have acquired during the initial phase of MBTI. This involves metacognitive shifts by relating to the problem of insomnia in a new or different way. It might also involve skillful action in thoughts and behaviors that do not directly involve trying to sleep, providing a different way to step outside of the territory of insomnia and reducing the attachment to wanting better sleep. On the basis of the metacognitive model of insomnia (Ong, Ulmer, & Manber, 2012), it directs the attention away from the nighttime symptoms and toward a more balanced and flexible perspective of insomnia with a commitment to broader values. The concept of seeing insomnia as a territory is borrowed from mindfulness-based cognitive therapy (MBCT), in which the territory of depression is used as a means of reconceptualizing areas to apply mindfulness skills to prevent the relapse of depression (Segal, Williams, & Teasdale, 2002).

The territory of insomnia might not be an intuitive concept that participants can immediately understand. Therefore, it is helpful to have a group discussion when explaining this concept. Instructors can begin by asking participants questions related to insomnia to determine whether there are any changes in their conceptualization of insomnia at this point in the MBTI program. Possible questions include the following:

- What does insomnia mean to you?
- Has the meaning of insomnia changed since you started this program?
- Are there other areas in your life that you feel are related to insomnia?

It might be helpful to distribute a handout with the criteria for insomnia disorders as a tool for discussion. Sometimes, drawing the territory of insomnia on a blackboard or whiteboard and having participants comment on what things fall into the different categories can aid in connecting the concept with the participant's experiences. The drawing usually consists of a series of concentric circles, with sleep disturbance at the core and the outer rings representing other domains or aspects of the experience of insomnia (see Figure 7.1). The key point to communicate in this discussion is that the experience of insomnia can include many areas outside of the symptoms of insomnia, such as feelings of isolation, loss of confidence, urgency to fix the problem, or changes in social schedule. Allowing each individual to discover what falls under his or her territory of insomnia can provide a more comprehensive map of different territories to work on that might be outside of sleeping at night. Following the larger group discussion, participants can break into small groups or partners to have more intimate discussions about what the territory of insomnia means for each participant. Specifically, participants should be asked to consider two questions: (a) What is your territory of insomnia? (b) How might you approach this territory in a mindful way?

HOMEWORK FOR SESSION 5

The homework for Session 5 is to alternate between a movement meditation (mindful walking, yoga) and a quiet meditation (sitting meditation, body scan) for at least 30 minutes per day, 6 days per week. Participants should also continue with their sleep consolidation and sleep reconditioning program based on any adjustments made during this session. Finally, participants should continue to log their activities into the sleep and meditation diary.

FIGURE 7.1

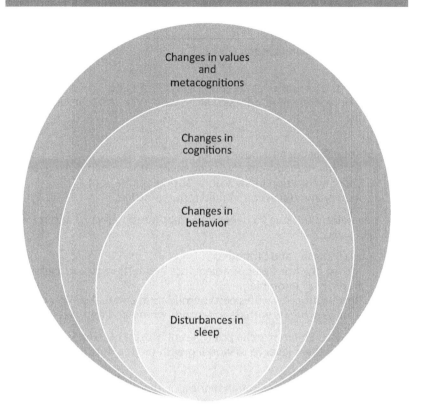

Changes in values
and
metacognitions

Changes in
cognitions

Changes in
behavior

Disturbances in
sleep

The territory of insomnia. This picture is an example of
how the "territory of insomnia" grows as the impact of
sleep disturbance extends into other domains. In drawing
the territory of insomnia, MBTI instructors should use specific examples from participants in each domain. This illustration can serve as a reminder that it is possible to work
on other layers of the territory of insomnia besides sleep.

Session 6: Acceptance and Letting Go

The major theme for Session 6 is to reinforce the concepts of working
with thoughts and feelings in the territory of insomnia, with a particular
emphasis on the principles of acceptance and letting go. The meditation
practice and period of inquiry follow the same structure as in previous
sessions. One variant that can be introduced during this session is to

---

EXHIBIT 7.2

Session 6 Outline

Theme: Acceptance and Letting Go

Objectives
1. Reinforce the principles of acceptance and letting go.
2. Explain how to use mindfulness skills to work with thoughts and feelings in the territory of insomnia.

Activities
1. Meditation Practice and Inquiry
   a. Movement meditation (walking meditation or mindful movement and stretching)
   b. Quiet meditation (body scan or sitting meditation)
   c. Inquiry and discussion of meditation practices

   Key Point: Continue to deepen the meditation practice and reinforce the mindfulness principles.

2. Insomnia Didactics and Strategies
   a. Review the principles of acceptance and letting go and make connection with the territory of insomnia.
   b. Review progress with sleep consolidation and make alterations as needed.
   c. Review progress with sleep reconditioning and reinforce instructions as needed.

   Key Points: Emphasize the principles of acceptance and letting go as metacognitive shifts and the relevance to working with the territory of insomnia.

Homework for Session 6
1. Complete sleep and meditation diaries.
2. Choice of meditation (mindful walking, yoga, sitting meditation, or body scan) for at least 6 days (30 minutes per day).
3. Continue with sleep consolidation and sleep reconditioning instructions.

---

invite participants to bring in a difficult thought, emotion, or body sensation to work with during the quiet meditation. This variant can be done to highlight the concepts of acceptance and letting go, the major theme of this session. This can be very challenging for participants as most might feel that the meditation is supposed to cultivate positive emotions and find that bringing in a negative thought or sensation is undesirable. If this arises, the period of inquiry can be used to explore different ways to work with thoughts or sensations that are normally judged to be negative (e.g., pain, anxiety, depressed thoughts). See Exhibit 7.2 for the Session 6 outline.

ACCEPTANCE AND LETTING GO

The didactic portion of Session 6 is focused on the mindfulness principles of acceptance and letting go. These are two very important principles to cultivate and keep alive while working with negative emotional reactions in response to sleep disturbance. Thus far, participants have only been instructed to practice these principles during meditations; how these principles can apply to the context of insomnia and how they can be used to work with the territory of insomnia have not been discussed. The reason for coming back to this concept at a later point in MBTI is that the practice of acceptance and letting go can be very challenging, and I have found that it is generally more helpful to allow participants the opportunity to engage in their own meditation practice for a period of time before focusing on acceptance and letting go. Furthermore, these principles can be very helpful for participants who are practicing meditations at home and following the sleep consolidation and sleep reconditioning instructions but not seeing any significant improvements in their sleep or daytime functioning. The principles of acceptance and letting go can serve as reminders of how to respond in a mindful way when improvements are not happening as quickly as desired.

The principle of letting go, or letting be, is actually inherent in many of the meditation practices. For example, in the body scan we bring attention to each area of the body and then let go of that area, bringing our attention to the next body area. This is essentially a practice of bringing attention to an area and then intentionally allowing the attention to move to another area without judging or becoming engaged in problem solving of that area. Another example is paying attention to the breath. Each exhalation is a practice of breathing out and letting go of that breath. In the context of insomnia, sleep naturally unfolds by letting go of conscious activities or of trying to control thoughts in the mind. In other words, one has to be ready to let go of being awake. This means letting go of the problems and pleasures that occur during the day to allow for sleep to happen.

One important distinction to make is that letting go is not pushing away thoughts or clearing the mind. In mindfulness practices, we are not trying to empty the mind or prevent thoughts from occurring. Attempts to do so are fruitless because the mind will always find something to latch onto. Instead, letting go is a way to allow thoughts to be as they are and to allow them to run their course. When thoughts are intentionally allowed to come in and out of conscious awareness without engagement, they are likely to eventually subside. This might seem like a counterintuitive approach to just allow thoughts to be present rather than to make them go away, but this is what happens when one is a trainspotter of the mind. Instructors might want to conduct a trainspotting meditation to help reinforce this message.

The principle of acceptance is also very important when working mindfully with the territory of insomnia. Although it might seem reasonable to expect that using the tools learned thus far should result in sleep improvements, sometimes the improvements do not happen as quickly as desired. As one might have noticed, the brain is quite a resilient organ and it still allows us to function even if we have been sleeping very little. Accepting that sleep may not happen exactly when desired, or for as long as we would like, is a key component of working with the territory of insomnia. At night, it can serve as a reminder to get out of bed when the mind and the body are not yet ready for sleep. During the day, accepting that we do not always function at full alertness can help to reduce the distress that might otherwise be an automatic reaction to little sleep.

One question that frequently arises during the discussion on acceptance is whether it is a passive way of "giving up," or a resignation to the idea that one has no control over the problem. If this comes up, instructors should remind participants that it is actually the opposite: Rather than giving up, one is making a conscious decision to accept or embrace what is happening. The difference is that mindful acceptance is an intentional choice, whereas giving up is a forced choice. One is choosing to actively respond by allowing or letting the feeling or experience happen rather than automatically avoiding, fixing, or being at the mercy of the unpleasant feeling. This shift toward an active approach can lead to new observations of the experience—that is, the negative emotions really were not as bad as originally perceived, and urgent action is not required. The key points are that it is not always helpful to try to fix or solve things and that the urge to fix something often adds a layer of stress. Acceptance provides another way to relate to the problem. This metacognitive shift often leads to a deeper understanding of the problem and allows creative solutions to emerge.

In a previously published article (Ong & Sholtes, 2010), my colleague and I described a case study of one participant in an MBTI program who had a breakthrough during the Session 6 discussion on acceptance and letting go. The patient was struggling to clear her mind at night and was frustrated that these thoughts kept returning. The dialogue that follows was adapted from Ong and Sholtes (p. 1188) and provides an example of how a therapist can lead the discussion on letting go and acceptance.

Participant 1: I still don't get how letting go works. During my meditations, I have been trying to clear my mind and sometimes I can keep it blank for a while but it always seems to come back.

Participant 2: Yes, I have that same problem. No matter how hard I try to let go, it keeps coming back. Then I feel like I am doing something wrong.

Instructor: So it sounds like there is effort to make the thoughts go away.

Participant 1: Yes, and if my mind keeps running around, then it is difficult to just say to myself, "accept this." It's

like I can't control anything and then just saying
forget it!

Instructor: I wonder what it might be like to work with these
thoughts in another way. Rather than using effort
to force these thoughts out, what if you just
allowed them to be.

Participant 1: Then they certainly won't go anywhere, and I'll be
in the same place.

Instructor: Perhaps, or you might find that the same thoughts
that keep coming back will sometimes go away on
their own. They might eventually find their way
back too! In other words, thoughts will come and
go, but forcing it to go in one direction is like trying
to reverse the flow of a powerful river.

Participant 1: So you are asking me not to try to clear my mind
of these thoughts?

Instructor: I am asking you to see what happens when you
just let your thoughts run their course. Rather
than trying to block or reverse the flow of a river,
try standing on the bank of the river. It is not the
thoughts you are trying to control, but instead it is
letting go of the effort of forcing these thoughts to
go in a certain direction.

Participant 1: Hmm . . . that's different than what I've been doing.

Participant 2: I never quite saw it that way either, but I'm starting
to see what you are talking about.

Instructor: See what happens when you practice letting go
of your *desire* to clear your thoughts in this way
during your meditations this week. Every time
the thoughts come back is another opportunity to
practice letting go!

In this discussion, the instructor reinforces the principles of acceptance
and letting go by gently encouraging the participant to try a different
way to work with her thoughts. The analogy of trying to stop the flow
of a river as opposed to standing on the bank of the river is one way to
help participants gain insight about the difference between letting go
and trying to clear the mind.

During the period of discussion of these two principles, instructors should ask participants to discuss one or more of these questions:
(a) What do you think people with insomnia avoid? (b) Why do we
cling to thoughts or behaviors that we would rather change? Practicing
the trainspotting exercise or reading the poem "The Guest House" from
Rumi (Barks, 1995) are also ways to engage participants and reinforce
the concepts of letting go and acceptance. This poem is also read in
MBSR and MBCT and serves as an excellent example of how inviting
all guests, good and bad, can be a wonderful and enriching experience.
Practicing the principles of letting go and acceptance are examples of

the metacognitive shift that can allow one to work with the outer layers of the territory of insomnia.

HOMEWORK FOR SESSION 6

Following the discussion on acceptance and letting go, instructors should allow participants 10 to 15 minutes to review and discuss the sleep consolidation schedules and sleep reconditioning program in small groups. Troubleshooting and discussions should be handled similar to Session 5. For the Session 6 homework, participants should continue with their sleep program, incorporating any adjustment to their schedule or instructions on the basis of the discussion. They can also practice their choice of meditation (quiet or movement) for at least 30 minutes per day, 6 days out of the week.

Session 7: Revisiting the Relationship With Sleep

Session 7 continues the theme of metacognitive shifting by bringing attention to the relationship with sleep and the concept of self-compassion. An activity called the *nurturing/depleting activity* is introduced as part of the discussion of self-compassion and self-care. This offers participants another way to manage energy and fatigue during the daytime that is not directly related to sleep at night. In addition, informal meditations are discussed as a means to incorporate mindfulness practices into daily life. The 3-minute breathing space is a brief, informal meditation that participants can use outside of a formal meditation practice. See Exhibit 7.3 for the Session 7 outline.

MEDITATION AND PERIOD OF INQUIRY

Earlier, I discussed the progression of how quiet meditations are first introduced to bring awareness to the mind and body while being still. Next, I introduced movement meditations to bring awareness to the mind and body in motion. Whereas formal meditations involve setting aside 30 minutes from everyday tasks to practice the meditations, informal meditations involve bringing mindfulness principles into everyday tasks. This includes practicing mindful eating, mindful exercising, mindful parenting, and even mindful working. This is the "end-game" of mindfulness practice; that is, it entails bringing the principles of mindfulness into

EXHIBIT 7.3

Session 7 Outline

Theme: Revisiting the Relationship With Sleep

Objectives
1. Revisit the relationship with sleep.
2. Discuss self-compassion and self-care in the context of insomnia.
3. Encourage ways to incorporate informal mindfulness practices into daily life.

Activities
1. Meditation Practice and Inquiry
    a. Movement meditation (walking meditation or mindful movement and stretching)
    b. Quiet meditation (body scan or sitting meditation)
    c. Inquiry and discussion of meditation practices, focusing on informal meditations
    d. Introduce the 3-minute breathing space

    Key Point: Encourage participants to begin the transition to broadening the meditation practice to include informal practices and to begin establishing a long-term plan for meditation practice.

2. Insomnia Didactics and Strategies
    a. Discuss the relationship with sleep as a metacognitive shift.
    b. Introduce the nurturing/depleting activities exercise as an act of self-compassion and self-care.
    c. Review progress with sleep consolidation and make alterations as needed.
    d. Review progress with sleep reconditioning and reinforce instructions as needed.

    Key Points: Revisit the relationship with sleep as a metacognitive shift. Use the nurturing/depleting activity to discover activities that are nurturing and activities that are depleting.

Homework for Session 7
1. Complete sleep and meditation diaries.
2. Choice of meditation with no guidance or CD for at least 6 days (30 minutes per day).
3. Continue with sleep consolidation and sleep reconditioning instructions.

our lives so that we are truly connecting with the moment-to-moment experience of living. Recall that in Session 1 (see Chapter 5), the eating meditation was the first meditation that was introduced in MBTI. After practicing formal meditations for several weeks, participants are brought back to informal meditation practices to help maintain mindfulness skills in their everyday living after the program.

In Session 7, instructors should reduce the formal meditation to about 20 minutes each, saving some time to introduce informal meditations. The 3-minute breathing space is an informal meditation that can be easily taught and can provide a structure for a brief meditation to ground oneself in the present moment. This "mini-meditation" was developed by Segal, Williams, and Teasdale (2002) as part of the MBCT program.

This informal meditation can gently bring attention to the breath and the current mental and physical state in three steps, each of which only takes about 1 minute. The purpose of the breathing space is to become grounded in the moment when we notice that acute stress is present or we notice that we are operating in automatic pilot mode. Gaining present-moment focus during times of stress or negative events puts one in a better position to take mindful action rather than make mindless reactions.

As described in Exhibit 7.4, the first minute is spent cultivating present-focused awareness. This allows one to acknowledge and register the experience with whatever is present—pleasant or unpleasant experiences. The second minute is spent gathering and redirecting attention to the breath. Attention is intentionally brought to the process of breathing to cultivate full awareness of the breath. The third minute is spent expanding the field of awareness to the body as a whole. This might include the posture, facial expression, or physical sensations in the body. If discomfort or pain is present, the participant can be encouraged to just bring attention to that area and allow it to be, practicing the principle of letting go and acceptance. After approximately 3 minutes, the awareness is brought back to what the person was previously doing.

One point of emphasis is that the breathing space is meant to cultivate mindfulness during stressful times. It is not meant to be used as an "escape hatch" to avoid the problem, nor is it meant to make one "feel

---

EXHIBIT 7.4

The 3-Minute Breathing Space

Notes: This brief meditation consists of three components (awareness, gathering and redirecting attention, expanding attention), each lasting approximately one minute.

Instructions:
1. Begin by having participants bring awareness to the present moment by adopting an erect and dignified posture.
2. Have participants close their eyes, if they choose. They may also do this meditation with their eyes open.
3. During the first minute, allow participants to acknowledge and register whatever thoughts, feelings, and sensations arise. Instructors can use prompts such as, *What thoughts are present? What feelings are here? What bodily sensations are we noticing?*
4. During the second minute, have participants gather and redirect attention to their breathing. Have participants note the sensations associated with each inhalation and exhalation.
5. During the third minute, encourage participants to expand the field of awareness around breathing so that it includes a sense of the body as a whole. This might include posture, facial expressions, pain, or other thoughts. If there are areas of pain or discomfort, encourage participants to bring attention to that area and just be present with those sensations.
6. End the meditation by ringing the chimes or bell. Or, instruct participants to open their eyes.

---

better" about the current situation—mindfulness is not about creating positive emotions. Instead, it is a self-regulatory tool that can bring us back to the platform of awareness so that we can put ourselves in a position to take mindful action.

Besides the 3-minute breathing space, other informal meditations can include the raisin-eating meditation or even drinking water mindfully. Wine tasting is another good example of how mindfulness principles can be brought into an activity that many people engage in as part of their lives. In wine tasting, attention is brought to each of our senses as we bring awareness to the experience of the wine so that we can perceive and enjoy the qualities. Mindful running or jogging can include bringing qualities of mindful walking to a faster pace. In MBTI, there are no specific limits or activities for introducing informal meditations. Typically, in Session 7 there is a discussion in small groups or between partners in which each group or dyad discusses how mindfulness can be practiced informally and each participant develops a plan to practice informal meditations at home.

RELATIONSHIP WITH SLEEP

When participants first begin MBTI, some describe a difficult relationship with sleep. I have heard some insomnia patients describe sleep as an "enemy" and that somehow, an activity they used to trust like a best friend has suddenly turned on them. This indicates that the relationship with sleep has changed. The didactic portion of Session 7 begins by having each participant reevaluate his or her relationship with sleep. This is another opportunity to reinforce the theme of metacognitive awareness and metacognitive shifts because the way one relates to sleep is not simply a function of thoughts and behaviors.

There are several principles that can be brought into this discussion. First, the principle of nonjudging allows us to see sleeplessness as a state rather than an enemy. If sleeplessness is present during the time in bed, this can be acknowledged, and there are different tools that we can use to work with sleeplessness. We can use beginner's mind to relearn how to approach each night with a fresh perspective, free of expectations. We can use the principle of letting go of expectations about sleep or desired amount of sleep to recognize that sleep needs might change, from night-to-night, as well as across the lifespan. By practicing the principle of acceptance when sleeplessness occurs, we can learn to work with it rather than trying to avoid it, which only elevates arousal and anxiety about sleep.

There is a poem by Billy Collins (2001) called "Insomnia" that I sometimes read to the group. This poem provides an interesting perspective of someone who describes a racing mind that will not stop. He states that "someone inside me will not get off his tricycle, will not stop tracing the same tight circle" and describes him as a "schoolboy in an ill-fitting jacket." This poem serves to illustrate a metacognitive shift such that the inability to fall asleep remains, but the speaker is able to work on the outer layers of the territory of insomnia and reduce secondary arousal. The verbs and adjectives used in the poem reflect how the person is able to stand back and just observe and describe rather than get engaged and frustrated. It is always interesting to listen to how a group of people with chronic insomnia react to this poem. Some feel that this is impossible to do, whereas others identify with the problem but do not think that just watching the mind race will help them fall asleep. This can create discussion points that remind participants about the practices of beginner's mind, letting go, and acceptance.

In the group discussion about the relationship with sleep, the instructor should ask participants about any changes they might have noticed in their relationship with sleep. Some comments I have heard from participants include the following:

- "Before, it was like I was wrestling in bed."
- "I don't feel like I am fighting with sleep anymore, even if it isn't the way I want."
- "I take life from a different perspective. For example, whether I have a good night or not, it [stress] is not there anymore. For example, it's 3:00 a.m. and I am awake. So what?"

Not everyone will report changes, and some participants might not totally understand the concept of the relationship with sleep. Sometimes this can be reframed as the attachment to sleep or the need to fix sleep. As before, MBTI instructors should be careful not to inadvertently give more attention or show preference to group members who report positive changes in their relationship with sleep.

SELF-COMPASSION AND THE NURTURING/ DEPLETING ACTIVITY

Self-compassion is an important tenet in Buddhist philosophy, but its role in mindfulness-based therapies has been debated (Hölzel et al., 2011). Typically, self-compassion is taught as an implicit part of doing meditations, but some scholars feel that self-compassion is a separate concept. For most mindfulness-based therapies, the act of practicing mindfulness meditation is an act of self-compassion because one is taking the time to bring focus to the mind and body and is thus an act of self-care. The openness and safe space created during the meditation practice and during the period of inquiry can also promote self-compassion.

In MBTI, self-compassion is seen as arising from the elements of taking a new metacognitive stance, including balance, flexibility, equanimity, and commitment to values. In addition to being implicitly taught during meditation practices, it is explicitly used during the nurturing/ depleting exercise, an activity that was adapted from MBCT (Segal, Williams, & Teasdale, 2002). This exercise is designed to allow participants to examine their daily lives and develop awareness of the type of activities that are nurturing and the types of activities that are depleting. This is done by creating an inventory of the energy transactions that occur during daily routines. By improving awareness of these energy transactions, participants can act with more self-compassion and self-care. This activity can be particularly important if daytime fatigue is present after several nights of poor sleep. Recall from Chapter 6 that fatigue involves an interpretation of the mental and physical energy available or the degree to which it takes energy to engage in an activity. Feeling fatigued often has negative feelings attached to it, so when this is present, one way to work mindfully with this is to take time to do more nurturing activities. These activities can help one to make a metacognitive shift by working with the interpretation of the energy available without changing the actual level of energy. Therefore, the nurturing/depleting activity complements the sleep consolidation and sleep reconditioning program by offering a direct tool for managing daytime fatigue.

The instructions for the nurturing/depleting activity are simple and involve three steps (see the Appendix, Handout 8). First, participants are asked to list, in as much detail as possible, all activities that they do during a typical day. They are then asked to review each activity and assign it a value of "N" if it is nurturing or "D" if it is depleting. Some activities might be both, depending on the day. In these cases, participants should decide on the basis of how they typically feel after engaging in the activity. Finally, participants are asked to tally the total number of Ns and Ds that are listed.

Once participants are done, the instructor asks one or two participants to read out loud the activities and to note whether the activity was an N or a D. Then they are asked to report the total number of Ns and Ds. The instructor should then lead a discussion based on the following questions:

1. Where is your energy going?
2. Of the Ns: How might you change things so that you can make more time to do these or become more aware of them?
3. Of the Ds: How might these activities be done less often?

In the discussion, it is usually noted that some of the same activities can be nurturing or depleting so that a different approach to the same activity might be considered nurturing rather than depleting. Instructors might consider discussing sleep specific examples: "trying" to nap can be depleting, whereas resting or meditating for the same amount of time can be refreshing. Once again, we are working to bring mindful attention to increase the range of responses to the experience of being fatigued. It also promotes a metacognitive shift away from the attachment to sleep by demonstrating to participants that there are other ways to work with daytime fatigue, even if they might be caused by insufficient sleep.

HOMEWORK FOR SESSION 7

Session 7 should end by having participants break into small groups or pairs to discuss their sleep program and homework practice for the last 15 to 20 minutes. The homework for Session 7 includes a choice of meditation with no guidance from digital media for at least 6 days out of the week. This is in preparation for developing a routine to continue the meditation practice after the end of the MBTI program. In addition, participants are asked to practice the 3-minute breathing space at least once per day, 6 days per week. Participants should continue to record their activities in the sleep and meditation diary and to continue with their sleep program, making any adjustments that were discussed during this session.

Bringing MBTI to Closure and Mindfulness to Life

8

M uch like any graduation, bringing mindfulness-based therapy for insomnia (MBTI) to closure is about preparing participants for the journey ahead. This chapter discusses the final session of MBTI and steps that instructors can take to prepare participants for maintaining mindfulness principles after MBTI has ended. I also discuss other meditations and activities that have been used in MBTI but are not considered to be core components. Finally, I discuss challenges and issues related to nonadherence, group dynamics, and homework assignments that instructors might face in delivering MBTI. For instructors, this is the end of MBTI, but for the participants, the journey for bringing mindfulness into their lives has just begun.

http://dx.doi.org/10.1037/14952-009

Mindfulness-Based Therapy for Insomnia, by J. C. Ong

Session 8: Living Mindfully After MBTI

Session 8 is the final session of MBTI, and the overall theme is to bring closure to the MBTI program and to prepare participants for keeping the mindfulness principles alive in their daily lives after MBTI. This includes reviewing participants' experiences in the class and setting up an action plan to continue the meditation practice. Instructors should also discuss how to work with future episodes of insomnia, should they arise. Many participants will have devoted considerable effort to practicing meditation during the past 8 weeks, and some might have openly shared emotions and vulnerable thoughts that have come up during their practice. Friendships might have developed between group members, and some people might have shared rides to the sessions. As a result, the final session can be an emotional experience for participants. Feelings of sadness that the group has to end may arise, or participants may have feelings of gratitude and joy for having a new set of tools to work with sleep problems and emotional distress. Even the instructor might have strong emotions that arise. Therefore, MBTI instructors should be prepared for the possibility of working with strong emotions during this last session. See Exhibit 8.1 for the Session 8 outline.

MEDITATION PRACTICE AND PERIOD OF INQUIRY

In leading the meditation practice for Session 8, instructors can shorten the practice to about 40 minutes, leaving more time for discussion. Instructors can also end with a sitting meditation to bring the formal practice in MBTI to a full circle, as this was the first formal practice that was taught in Session 1. During the period of inquiry, instructors should discuss how to continue a meditation practice beyond the end of the MBTI program. Information about meditation groups in the community or supporting materials (e.g., CDs, apps, websites) can be helpful. Participants should be encouraged to set short-term and long-term goals for meditation practice. Short-term goals might be the week-to-week goals of practicing at least 30 minutes per day, 6 days per week, much like the homework recommendations during MBTI. Long-term goals might include attending a meditation retreat once per year or joining a local meditation group. Occasionally, participants in the group are motivated to continue meeting and organize their own groups to continue practicing the principles learned during MBTI. The other point of discussion is to review what people have learned in the program. This is a good time to revisit the goals that participants were asked to set aside at the beginning of the MBTI program. Typically, each participant

---

EXHIBIT 8.1

Session 8 Outline

Theme: Living Mindfully After MBTI

Objectives
1. Provide guidance on mindfulness meditation (formal and informal) beyond this program
2. Set up an action plan for future episodes of insomnia.

Activities
1. Meditation Practice and Inquiry
   a. Sitting meditation with choiceless awareness
   b. Inquiry and discussion of meditation practices, focusing on how participants can establish a long-term practice
   c. Discussion on lessons learned during MBTI

   Key Point: Develop a short-term and long-term plan for continuing the meditation practice beyond MBTI. Review what participants have learned in MBTI.

2. Insomnia Didactics and Strategies
   a. Prepare participants for relapse prevention by putting together an action plan for insomnia.

   Key Point: Help participants develop an action plan to work with future episodes of insomnia.

3. Closing Ceremony
   a. Form a circle and encourage participants to share their experience in MBTI.

   Key Point: Provide a sense of closure to the program and encouragement for participants to continue in their own journey.

---

is asked two questions: (a) Has anything changed for you since the start of the MBTI program? and (b) Is there anything you have discovered in practicing mindfulness meditation?

AN ACTION PLAN FOR INSOMNIA

Following the period of inquiry, the insomnia-related didactic component of the final session addresses relapse prevention and strategies for dealing with future episodes of insomnia, should they arise. Because insomnia is a condition that can occur in bouts, it is likely that participants will encounter future bouts of sleep disturbance, especially during periods of stress. Therefore, it is particularly helpful to have an action plan ready ahead of the recurrence of insomnia, which will remind participants how to use the tools that they accumulated during the MBTI program.

During this activity, instructors should help each participant put together such an action plan. First, instructors should lead a general

discussion on some possible ways to work with future episodes of insomnia using what they have learned during the MBTI program. If possible,
the instructor should write these on a blackboard or whiteboard so that
participants can see the entire list that has been generated by the group.
Then, participants can break into small groups or dyads to discuss their
own action plans to work with the territory of insomnia. They should
be given Handout 9 (see Appendix) so that they can generate their
own action plan. They can use anything from the group list, or other
things that they feel would be helpful. Subsequently, the large group is
reunited, and each participant is asked to describe his or her action plan
based on what they have written in Handout 9. If participants are stuck
or the instructor needs some ideas to help the group brainstorm, here
are some ideas to facilitate the discussion:

The first step is to become aware of what is going on.

1. Awareness of mental and physical states—Are you sleepy? Are
   you fatigued?
2. Awareness of sleep/wake patterns; keep a sleep diary.
3. Note what stressors are present during the day.
4. Are you reacting automatically to sleep disruption?
5. Are you avoiding unwanted wakefulness by going to bed?

The second step is to make a choice of how to respond.

1. Accept and let go.
2. Increase nurturing activities (especially if daytime fatigue seems
   to be a problem).
3. Choose to wake up at the same time.
4. Choose to follow sleep consolidation or sleep reconditioning
   instructions without judgment.
5. Choose to take a 3-minute breathing space to help cope with
   daytime stress.
6. Choose to take a nap if sensations of sleepiness are overwhelming.
7. Be a trainspotter of the mind.
8. Use the cloud metaphor as a meditation.

During the discussion, the instructor should reinforce the principles
of mindfulness and remind participants that the action plan should be
done with awareness and intention rather than automatic reactions in
an effort to regain sleep. Once each participant has completed Handout 9,
the final step is to determine what to do with the handout. Many participants decide to put the handout on their refrigerator or bulletin board.
Others have e-mailed the plan to themselves. Some have given it to
another group member and asked them to mail it to them in 6 months,
or some set amount of time. To be effective, the action plan should be in a
place that is accessible and easy to find in the future, if insomnia returns.

It should be noted that not all participants in a group will be in remission from insomnia. Hopefully, these individuals will have experienced some changes in their symptoms or some metacognitive shift regarding what insomnia means to them. For those still struggling with insomnia, the action plan can focus on continuing the MBTI activities. This can include a personal plan for continuing the meditation practice, the sleep consolidation program, and the sleep reconditioning program. The action plan might also include taking another look at the territory of insomnia after a certain period of time (e.g., every 2 weeks) to reexamine areas that the individual can work on. Instructors should commend these participants for completing MBTI (they could have easily dropped out when they did not see any progress) and provide encouragement for continuing the MBTI activities. It is possible for people to see improvements after MBTI, if they continue to implement the activities on their own. If the sleep problem persists, then a referral to a sleep disorders clinic is warranted for further evaluation.

CLOSING CEREMONY

The final activity in MBTI is a closing ceremony to provide a sense of closure to the program and to acknowledge the hard work and contributions of each participant. The ceremony can also encourage participants to continue on their own journey or stay connected to help each other in their journeys. There are many options for the closing ceremony. One that has worked very well is to have a closing circle in which the group gathers in a close circle in chairs or on the floor, and each participant takes turns sharing his or her experience in MBTI. The meditation bell (or chimes) that the instructor uses to close the meditation practice is then passed around to the participant who wishes to speak. After sharing, the participant then rings the bell and passes it to the next participant. Participants usually enjoy ringing the bell!

If participants are unsure about what to share, encourage them to think back to their original goals: What did you want/hope for? What did you get out of this program, if anything? Why did you stay? What did you learn? What are your biggest obstacles to growth and healing? What strategies might work to not get stuck? Some examples of what past participants have shared are as follows:

- "I learned that I don't have to go to bed!"
- "I feel like I have a new path in life. I have a more positive attitude about life and feel happier about who I am."
- "I feel like my depression improved. I also noticed that there are less distractions, like noise does not bother me as much."
- "I have improved self-confidence with new tools for dealing with frustration."

■ "I realized how much I think about outcomes and how attached I am to always striving to achieve. I guess I learned this from early schooling but this class helped me to 'unlearn this.' I'm very surprised at how relaxing and relieving this makes me feel. Never would have thought that it works this way."

It is interesting to note that these comments are about ways in which the participants' lives have changed rather than how sleep has changed. These are examples that are consistent with the shift toward a new metacognitive stance that is connected with broader values in life, not just fixing the sleep problem.

It is also possible to just practice mindful listening, so participants should not be forced to share anything. The instructor might also consider sharing first, to serve as an example. Some instructors share a feeling of deep gratitude for the participants' openness and willingness to engage and work hard. Also, some share an appreciation for the opportunity to share such a profoundly healing and beautiful practice with all of the group members. I have also found that providing a "certificate of compassion" (see Appendix, Handout 10) can provide a sense of accomplishment for participants. One participant even wanted his picture taken with me handing him his certificate of compassion to remind him of his efforts in MBTI!

Meditation Retreat

In addition to the eight weekly sessions, we have offered an all-day retreat as part of MBTI to further enhance the practice of meditation and to provide participants an opportunity to experience a deeper level of meditation practice. Similar to the format in mindfulness-based stress reduction (MBSR), the meditation retreat is usually held on a weekend between Sessions 6 and 7 and lasts for about 6 hours. For example, a typical retreat might occur on the Saturday between Sessions 6 and 7 from 9:00 a.m. to 3:00 p.m. (see Exhibit 8.2 for a sample schedule). After a brief welcome and introduction of the retreat day, the majority of the day is conducted in *noble silence*, a term used in meditation retreats. Noble silence refers to maintaining silence of verbal and nonverbal communication, including speech, body, and mind, providing a backdrop for practicing mindfulness. The purpose is to enhance the experience of meditation by bringing greater awareness to the present moment without distraction of verbal and nonverbal noise. After the concept of noble silence is introduced, the instructor guides participants through a number of meditation practices throughout the day. These practices typically include the ones already introduced during the pre-

EXHIBIT 8.2

Sample Meditation Retreat Schedule

Time	Practice/Activity
9:00–9:10 a.m.	Welcome and introduction
9:10–9:30 a.m.	Sitting meditation
9:30–10:00 a.m.	Mindful movement and yoga
10:00–10:10 a.m.	Break
10:10–10:30 a.m.	Body scan
10:30–11:00 a.m.	Walking meditation
11:00–11:30 a.m.	Sitting meditation
11:30 a.m.–12:30 p.m.	Lunch
12:30–12:45 p.m.	Sitting meditation/reflection
12:45–1:15 p.m.	Walking meditation
1:15–1:45 p.m.	Metta meditation
1:45–1:50 p.m.	Break
1:50–2:00 p.m.	Brief mindful movement
2:00–2:15 p.m.	Mindful sharing
2:15–2:45 p.m.	Group sharing and discussion
2:45–3:00 p.m.	Closing sitting meditation

vious sessions (e.g., sitting, body scan, walking, yoga), but instructors can introduce new meditations (e.g., lake or mountain meditation) or other forms of mindful movement (e.g., qi gong, tai chi) that extend the meditation practice. Typically, 20 to 30 minutes are set aside for each practice and participants are given two 10- to 15-minute breaks and a 1-hour lunch, which is conducted in silence.

Is the meditation retreat essential to MBTI? I have run MBTI groups with and without the meditation retreat. At times, I have coordinated the retreat with an MBSR class, which allowed for a larger, more diverse group that is more common in meditation retreats. I have also invited past graduates of MBTI to attend the meditation retreat. At this point, I do not have data to support whether or not the retreat makes a difference. Anecdotally, participants generally find the retreat to be a positive experience that enhances their understanding of mindfulness. Some find it to be a unique and very powerful experience, whereas others find it to be marginally helpful. Many people have strong reactions to the concept of noble silence. A frequent comment is how difficult it is to go 5 to 6 hours without communicating, especially in today's society of mobile technology. Because this is something that cannot be replicated in a session, it indicates that the meditation retreat can be a valuable experience in learning and practicing mindfulness principles.

My recommendation is to include the meditation retreat as part of MBTI if at all possible. If there are other mindfulness-based programs in the local area, it might be possible to coordinate a day-long retreat with other groups, as we have done in the past. I would also recommend that the decision to have the retreat should be made prior to starting MBTI so that instructions about the date and time of the retreat are given at the beginning of the program. In one MBTI group, the decision to hold a retreat was not finalized until after the program started, and therefore the date and time were not announced until the third session. As a result, several participants were not able to make it and the turnout was very low. Finally, it should be emphasized that many people find the retreat to be a unique and powerful experience, so it is a rare opportunity to go a full day without communicating.

Reflections on Delivering MBTI

The outline, activities, and scripts presented in this section of the book are intended to provide guidance to those who are interested in bringing mindfulness meditation and its principles to help people who suffer from chronic insomnia. These activities were informed by my own training in psychology—behavioral sleep medicine, MBSR, and mindfulness-based cognitive therapy—and should not be considered the "right way." There are many ways to teach mindfulness principles and practices to people with chronic insomnia. Instructors should not feel limited by the structure but should feel free to adapt this structure to include other activities, techniques, or meditations, so long as these are grounded in the principles and practices of mindfulness. In the following paragraphs, I describe other activities that are not part of the core MBTI program but that can be considered optional activities that instructors might want to include, if they feel they are appropriate. I also reflect on various challenges I encountered in teaching MBTI. The reader can consider this section to be my "process notes" on the lessons learned by leading MBTI groups.

LOVING-KINDNESS MEDITATION (METTA MEDITATION)

At times, I have experimented with different meditation practices. For example, I sometimes lead a loving-kindness, or Metta meditation, in Session 7 to facilitate the discussion about self-compassion (see Stahl & Goldstein, 2010). This is particularly useful if the meditation retreat is held between Sessions 6 and 7 and the Metta meditation is first introduced during the retreat. The Metta meditation is somewhat different from the other meditations in MBTI, where the focus of attention is on mindful awareness. During a Metta meditation, the focus of attention is brought to cultivating compassion. This is done by repeating a series of phrases reflecting compassion, starting with the attention on the self:

1. May I be safe.
2. May I be healthy.
3. May I be at ease (or free from harm).
4. May I be at peace.

The reason for starting with the self is to acknowledge the possibility that acts of kindness and benevolence can be cultivated with practice and this practice begins by treating the self with compassion. After leading the group through these first four phrases, the instructor leads the group through a series of progressive steps using these phrases. After the self, the compassion should be directed toward benefactors, such as a family member, a mentor, or an individual who has made a significant impact. Here, the phrases might be

1. May (benefactor) be safe.
2. May (benefactor) be healthy.
3. May (benefactor) be at ease (or free from harm).
4. May (benefactor) be at peace.

The phrases of compassion are then repeated for an acquaintance, or someone with a neutral or casual connection. The next step is to repeat the phrases for an enemy. This can be very difficult, and participants might wonder why we would want to cultivate compassion toward someone that we dislike. The purpose of this is to practice compassion for all human beings regardless of our attachment to the type of relationship we have with that person. This step might be too challenging for some people. If that is the case, the participant can be directed to repeat the phrases of compassion toward a benefactor with whom they have been angry or had a recent conflict. Finally, the phrases of compassion are repeated for all beings.

1. May all beings be safe.
2. May all beings be healthy.
3. May all beings be at ease (or free from harm).
4. May all beings be at peace.

Some participants comment that the Metta meditation feels like a prayer or something more spiritual since the phrases include a wish or desire for benevolence, which is different from the other meditations. Although it should be acknowledged that this meditation is not specifically a practice of mindful awareness, the concept of self-compassion is an aspect of mindfulness and requires practice. The series of steps is meant to spread out the compassion and to practice directing compassion at others. In practicing the Metta meditation, some people may experience self-hatred, the opposite feeling of self-compassion. If this occurs, instructors should normalize the experience and emphasize that there is nothing wrong if this comes up. Because this is a rather challenging meditation, it is best to introduce this toward the end of the program. Alternatively, this meditation can be left out if the instructor feels that introducing these concepts and this meditation would confuse participants. MBTI instructors should use their judgment to determine their own comfort level with leading a Metta meditation and also consider what is appropriate for each MBTI group.

COPING STRATEGIES

If participants seem to be having problems with stress management and time permits, instructors can integrate mindfulness principles with the coping strategies that are derived from stress management tools in psychotherapy and behavioral medicine (Lazarus & Folkman, 1984). According to Lazarus and Folkman (1984), there are two strategies for coping with stressful situations: problem-focused coping and emotion-focused coping. In *problem-focused coping*, the source of stress is first identified and if an immediate solution is possible, one works directly with the situation at hand by determining what actions need to be taken and what resources are available. In other situations, the problem cannot be changed or resources are not immediately available to solve the problem. In this situation, *emotion-focused coping* would be more appropriate. This strategy uses cognitive strategies to reframe the situation and work with thoughts and emotions about the situation. Both problem-focused and emotion-focused coping are very effective means of coping with daily stress and can be used together.

The approach taken in MBTI is very similar to the Lazarus and Folkman (1984) model of stress and coping. Recall that the first step in cultivating mindfulness is to become grounded in the present moment, noting mental and physical reactions to the situation. This could be done by engaging in a 3-minute breathing space or simply by directing attention to thoughts and feelings. Once the problem can be seen with clarity, free of the emotional reactions that might be habitually attached to the situation, then a more intentional, mindful response is now possible. Sometimes this might lead to a determination that is feasible to take steps to work with the problem. Other times, it might be possible to choose to work with thoughts and feelings, or it might be possible to accept these thoughts and feeling and just let then pass and see what happens. I have used this model during discussions in Session 7 about bringing mindfulness into our daily lives or during the nurturing/depleting activity.

WORKING WITH NONADHERENCE
AND PATIENT RESISTANCE

MBTI instructors should anticipate challenges related to nonadherence to homework or resistance from patients to implement the recommendations at home. In some cases, nonadherence is due to a failure to fully understanding the instructions of the homework or activity. If instructors begin to notice a pattern that either the group did not seem to complete the homework or that an individual repeatedly does not complete the homework, the instructor might consider asking specific questions to see if the instructions are clear. More frequently, the reason for nonadherence is lack of motivation or failure to embrace the rationale for the task.

Perhaps the most common area of nonadherence is keeping the scheduled sleep window as part of the sleep consolidation program. Patients will often decide against following their sleep window on some nights because they are "too tired," so they go to bed earlier at night or stay in bed later in the morning. In these situations, I ask why they did not follow the schedule and connect it with the attachment to outcomes (i.e., wanting more sleep). This can be helpful to illustrate why those behaviors are not likely to resolve their insomnia, even if they ended up sleeping more that night. Depending on what session this occurs, if the territory of insomnia has been introduced, this could provide another opportunity to revisit that patient's territory. MBTI instructors should gently offer participants the opportunity to discover what might happen if they let go of their attachment to wanting more sleep and simply follow the schedule. If they chose not to, instructors should suggest that the participant bring his or her attention to what arises at the moment when they decide not to follow the sleep schedule and see if their mental or physical state is congruent with their decision. Other group members can be helpful in processing nonadherence as they can talk about their struggles and successes with implementing the sleep consolidation instructions. Hearing these stories from other participants can help buy-in, as opposed to hearing encouragement from the instructor. As noted earlier, this should happen organically rather than directing group members to help others.

A second common area of nonadherence is with the sleep reconditioning instruction of getting out of bed when not sleepy. Many people will claim that it is too cold or undesirable to leave the bed in the middle of the night. Some will be afraid that getting up will decrease the chances of falling back to sleep. As in the case with nonadherence to sleep consolidation, asking patients for their reasons for not getting out of bed will very likely elicit a response that exemplifies an attachment to sleep or avoidance of wakefulness, driven by the fear that getting out of bed will reduce their chances of sleeping. This provides an opportunity to reinforce the importance of metacognitive shifting and letting go of the attachment. Again, mindful awareness of the mental and physical state should guide whether or one should follow the sleep reconditioning instructions. MBTI instructors should note if there are real safety concerns related to getting out of bed in the middle of the night for older adults or participants with mobility issues. In this scenario, the instructor might advise the participant to sit up in bed and get out of sleep mode.

One issue that can arise with practicing meditation is when a patient has previous experience with meditation, yoga, or mindfulness principles. I have encountered a few instances in which this can lead to making judgments about the way that meditation is taught in MBTI and some resistance to engaging in these practices. Typically, this becomes an issue of "my way" versus "your way" for the participant. Although there have been others who had a previous meditation practice and were able to remain open-minded about MBTI, this is an issue to be aware of when teaching mindfulness. When this has come up for me, I have gently encouraged the participant to practice beginner's mind and try following the meditation as it is taught in MBTI. Later, they can decide on their own if they wish to continue practicing the way that they were previously taught or to use the approach they learned in MBTI. I believe it is important to give participants the freedom to choose but to also encourage openness to trying something new.

Another form of nonadherence is poor attendance. At the beginning of the first session, I request that participants attend every class along with the meditation retreat and to let me know in advance if they cannot make any of the sessions. If possible, I offer some form of make-up when absences do occur. This could be over the phone to review sleep schedules or the meditation practice. I have also had patients come in early or stay late after a session to discuss what they missed. If participants miss a session without notification, I usually make an effort to contact them. Of course, some patients will drop out and never come back, but instructors should generally make efforts to maintain continuity with the MBTI materials in the event of absences. Staying in contact with participants and maintaining an openness for participants to choose whether or not they wish to continue with the program can promote rapport and decrease attrition.

MANAGING GROUP DYNAMICS AND SENSITIVE ISSUES

Because MBTI is designed to be delivered in groups, the dynamics among group members can play a role in the environment and tone during the sessions. As with any group situation, strong individual personalities can sometimes be dominant, making other group members feel timid or reluctant to participate. Occasionally, small cliques can also form, which can lead to some group members feeling excluded or minimized during discussions. This can have a detrimental effect on that individual and also impact the willingness to share during the period of inquiry. It is difficult to predict which group members will interact with or respond to each other, and personality differences can emerge. One way to minimize interference with group dynamics is to screen for obvious personality disorders during the pre-MBTI assessment that was discussed in Chapter 4.

In other cases, a group member might be very talkative and unintentionally dominate the period of inquiry because he or she has a lot to share. As mentioned before, the MBTI instructor should be responsible for creating a safe space for all participants to practice meditation and share their discoveries. If there are group members who are dominating the conversation or making judgments about other participant's actions, the instructor should first discuss this with the disruptive member privately. If the participant does not respond to this, then the MBTI instructor should consider the extent of the disruption and judge whether or not it is appropriate to remove the disruptive member.

Because strong emotions can arise during meditations, it is possible that a group member might share very sensitive information and become emotional, either during the meditation or during the period of inquiry. If appropriate, MBTI instructors should assess the emotional status of the group member and discuss possible referrals or assess any safety issues. Although there are no specific exclusion criteria for MBTI, those who have unstable medical or psychiatric conditions might not be capable of practicing mindfulness meditation. If sensitive information is shared with other group members, the MBTI instructor should remind all participants about maintaining group confidentiality and not to discuss the sensitive information outside of the group (see Chapter 5). Psychologists may wish to review the American Psychological Association (APA) *Ethical Principles of Psychologists and Code of Conduct* (APA, 2010) regarding privacy and confidentiality if issues arise within a group. Other professionals should consult with their own professional code of conduct or governing organization for further guidance.

Lack of improvement or impatience can also impact the MBTI group. Usually, at least one or two group members will show some improvement within the first 2 to 3 weeks. When these group members share their experiences, it can motivate the others to continue with their practice, even if they have not yet seen any direct benefits. When none of the group members are seeing any benefits within the first few weeks, it can lead to skepticism about the approach and decrease morale. As with the personality issues, it is difficult to predict who will respond to MBTI and how quickly a patient will respond. Even if none of the members in an MBTI group are reporting changes to their sleep, it is recommended to reinforce the message of nonjudging and letting go of goals and to continue with the practice. I have never had an MBTI group where not a single participant was able to identify at least some changes to their symptoms by the end of the program.

INTERPERSONAL ASPECTS OF DELIVERING MBTI

Given the issues related to resistance and group dynamics, I have been surprised at the sparse literature and limited discussion about the interpersonal aspects of working with insomnia patients. At the Stanford Sleep Clinic, we conducted a study examining therapeutic alliance in group cognitive behavior therapy for insomnia that was led by Dr. Michael Constantino (see Constantino et al., 2007). The study found that patients who perceived their therapist as being critically confrontative were more likely to drop out of treatment. These individuals were also more likely to have poorer treatment outcomes if they also had high expectations about treatment. Overall, the findings indicated that cognitive behavior therapy for insomnia was most effective when the therapeutic relationship comprised reciprocal exchanges that were affiliative, autonomy granting, and lacking in hostile control or critical confrontation. These qualities are consistent with a mindful stance that MBTI instructors are trained to embody.

Beyond treating insomnia, the importance of the therapist–patient interaction has been well-documented, particularly in the treatment of depression. McCullough (2003) developed a treatment program specifically for chronic depression, the cognitive behavioral analysis system of psychotherapy (CBASP). In CBASP, the therapist uses the interpersonal interaction in a disciplined and intentional way to allow patients to work through his or her problems. This requires a mature and experienced skill set and it is not recommended for novice therapists.

In MBTI, the role of the instructor is to lead the meditations, to facilitate the group discussions by creating a safe space for participants to discuss their experiences with other group members, and to provide instructions for implementing the behavioral strategies for insomnia at home. As noted earlier, participants in MBTI will sometimes share very sensitive, vulnerable experiences that might arise during meditations or during group discussions, and there is also a certain level of intimacy that typically evolves with the group. Similar to CBASP, MBTI instructors, ideally, should be experienced in working with vulnerable individuals and have the maturity to handle deeper levels of emotion that might arise during the intervention.

Another challenging aspect of delivering MBTI is to avoid trying to "fix" patients or show them the "right way" to do something.

For example, when leading the period of inquiry, it is important that instructors allow participants to share their experiences and describe their observations and changes without editing or judging. It can be difficult to refrain from using a comment as a "teaching point" to show the group how to do something "the right way" or even to show that something is a preferred way. However, by pointing out something as being "right," one sets the stage for identifying a preference for one way versus another, which is inconsistent with the principles of non-judging and nonattachment to outcomes. This is an important ongoing lesson that requires continued mindfulness practice and patience, trust, and awareness of the instructor's own reaction to stay mindful in leading the meditations and group discussions. In these situations, maintaining a mindful presence might require the instructor to simply acknowledge what is being said and to ask others for their reaction. This is where a strong personal commitment to mindfulness can be very helpful and allows an instructor to respond skillfully in these situations.

On the basis of my experiences, I have developed three key interpersonal principles for delivering MBTI:

1. *Be cognizant about trying to fix a patient's problems.* As previously noted, one of the important differences between a mindfulness-based approach and cognitive behavioral approaches is the importance of allowing patients to find their own way through a problem. In MBTI, people with insomnia are provided with the tools and framework for allowing sleep to come back, not for trying to make sleep happen.

2. *Embody a mindful stance that is composed, patient, and compassionate.* A mindful metacognitive stance is fostered by a personal meditation practice and knowledge of BSM. Patients will sometimes panic or become very distressed when they do not see improvements or if their sleep becomes worse again. In these situations, it is important as a therapist to maintain balance and equanimity, while communicating confidence that the patient can still find a way to work out of his or her sleep problem.

3. *Take a patient-centered approach.* In sports, a good coach gets the most out of the players by figuring how to put them in a position to succeed based on their skill sets. In a similar way, an MBTI instructor's job is to teach insomnia patients how to manage their behaviors, thoughts, and metacognitions such that they are in the best possible position to sleep. MBTI instructors should encourage patients to be their own "curious scientists" and elicit their discoveries along the way. This approach empowers patients to discover their own answers rather than have the instructor fix the problem for them.

CHALLENGES IN PRACTICING MEDITATION

Establishing a personal meditation practice can be very challenging, and many questions frequently come up during the first few sessions of MBTI. For example, what is the best time to meditate? There is no evidence of an ideal time to meditate. However, when starting out, it is best not to meditate in bed. For many people, meditating in the morning, shortly after waking up, or in the evening, when partners and children are not likely to disturb the meditation, are good guidelines. Ideally, the space to practice the meditation at home is private, but one does not have to have a meditation cushion or mat. Depending on the type of practice, meditation can be done on a chair, walking in circles, or even while stretching in a gym or exercise room.

Participants frequently complain that adding the meditation practice to their lives is one more thing to add to an already busy schedule. This should not be disputed, as meditation does take time and effort. However, participants should be reminded that meditation is not a hobby, job, or responsibility. It is a practice, and the practice leads to new skills, both mental and physical. If participants can take 30 minutes out of each day to practice meditation, they will be able to learn these skills. Some sacrifice might be needed, whether it is watching one less television show or spending 30 fewer minutes with the family. Or it might even be spending 30 fewer minutes in bed. In making these changes, participants might develop a greater awareness of resistance to change. Also, in making changes to the sleep schedule, most participants will be spending less time in bed. Therefore, the overall program might not yield any net loss in waking time.

SLEEP AND MEDITATION DIARIES

Every week, participants are asked to keep diaries on their sleep and meditation activities. Occasionally, a participant will become frustrated with this, especially if he or she is not seeing changes in their sleep patterns. Although keeping track of sleep and meditation is supposed to bring awareness to these activities, it can backfire for some individuals and lead to more stress. In these situations, I usually review the importance of keeping the diaries, but in the spirit of openness and discovery, I offer the option of seeing what happens if the diaries are not kept for 1 week and progress is reviewed verbally. Sometimes this can be helpful for participants to identify that they are still attached to the outcome of wanting to sleep better. Other times there is a sense of relief and this can serve as a breakthrough to facilitate their use of the other tools in the program. The decision of whether or not to allow participants the option of not completing diaries requires skillful judgment by the instructor, guided by experience and a sense of whether or not the resistance to keeping diaries is driven by a lack of motivation or by stress from keeping the diaries.

BEYOND SESSION 8

MBTI is designed as an 8-week program, and it is meant to serve as a starting point for bringing mindfulness into the lives of participants. At this point, we have not developed any formal follow-up programs or booster sessions to help participants continue their meditation practice or maintain their tools for working with insomnia. As mentioned earlier, we typically invite graduates of our past MBTI programs to attend the all-day retreat, which provides an opportunity for some to reignite or continue their meditation practice. MBTI instructors should also identify individuals who report serious symptoms of a mood or anxiety disorder and discuss possible referrals to a mental health practitioner for further help. It is possible that some participants might require further help with their sleep problems. In these cases, referrals should be made to a sleep specialist or sleep clinic for further evaluation. For some people, MBTI is just the first step in making changes to their lifestyle or addressing medical or psychiatric conditions that are related to their sleep problem.

MBTI IN THE LABORATORY AND THE REAL WORLD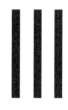

Is Mindfulness Meditation an Effective Treatment for Insomnia?

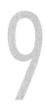

Part II of this book focused narrowly on the contents and delivery of the mindfulness-based therapy for insomnia (MBTI) program. Part III broadens the scope to examine the empirical evidence for using MBTI and other mindfulness and acceptance-based programs to treat insomnia and to consider how these interventions fit with other treatments that were discussed in Part I. The purpose of this section is to offer a perspective on how mindfulness-based treatment programs can be placed within the context of the current treatment options for insomnia and to provide ideas for future activities aimed at improving and disseminating MBTI. In this chapter, I describe the process of developing MBTI and the series of research studies that my colleagues and I have conducted in this area. In doing so, I elaborate on how we arrived at the current program and the considerations that led to deciding on the approach taken in MBTI. I also review the literature on other mindfulness-based interventions that have been used to improve sleep disturbance, and I discuss areas for future research. In Chapter 10, I offer my perspective on issues

http://dx.doi.org/10.1037/14952-010
Mindfulness-Based Therapy for Insomnia, by J. C. Ong

related to the delivery and dissemination of mindfulness-based treatment programs as a treatment for insomnia within the health care system.

Origins of MBTI

It is one thing to have a great idea for a new intervention. It is another thing to take that idea and design a research study that is rigorous enough to yield compelling findings. One study is insufficient to indicate that this new intervention is ready to be delivered to patients in clinics. An even greater challenge lies in having a long-term plan and vision to conduct a series of studies that will systematically provide evidence that the intervention works. These steps involve first testing the feasibility of the idea (i.e., proof of concept), then testing the intervention under controlled conditions (i.e., evidence of efficacy) and in real-world situations (i.e., evidence of effectiveness). Finally, the evidence needs to be compelling for practitioners to adopt the new intervention and for policymakers to accept the new intervention as a cost-effective tool within the health care system.

Developing and testing a treatment takes considerable time and often involves an iterative process of refinement. There is an established process for pharmacological treatments that typically takes at least 8 to 12 years between the time a drug is developed in the laboratory and when it receives approval by the U.S. Food and Drug Administration (Lipsky & Sharp, 2001). In contrast, there are no established standards for developing behavioral or meditation-based treatments. Although some models for behavioral treatment development have been proposed (Ong, Wickwire, Southam-Gerow, Schumacher, & Orsillo, 2008; Rounsaville, Carroll, & Onken, 2001), the process of treatment development receives much less attention compared with the outcome data. Furthermore, the lessons learned by the investigators along the way often come from clinical observations, anecdotes, or feedback from participants that do not get published. Therefore, it is rare that the story of how a treatment was developed ever gets told.

The following sections provide a summary of the research we have conducted on MBTI. Although many of the quantitative findings can be found in the referenced publications, I also add some commentary about how and why we made certain decisions to provide a context for understanding our study design and the implications of our findings. I believe that this part of the story is important because it provides an understanding of how the various components of MBTI came together as a program.

Treatment Development:
Proof-of-Concept Testing

When we first identified the need to develop an insomnia treatment that used mindfulness meditation, we recruited the help of Dr. Shauna Shapiro, a professor at Santa Clara University who is an expert in mindfulness-based programs and who had previously published on mindfulness and sleep disturbances. Because cognitive behavior therapy for insomnia (CBT-I) was already available as a treatment option, we wanted to make sure that our new intervention had distinct features. Mindfulness meditation was a novel treatment for insomnia, but we were unsure how people with insomnia would react if we were to ask them to meditate. Would they think that we were going to "meditate them to sleep"? Would this come across as some strange "new age" or "alternative" treatment that would not be appealing to a broad audience? Would they think this is too much work and refuse to come back? With these questions and concerns in the back of our mind, we set out to conduct a preliminary study to test our concept.

Our initial thought in putting together a treatment package using mindfulness meditation was to simply replace the cognitive component with mindfulness and add it to the main behavioral components of CBT-I, which include sleep restriction, stimulus control, and sleep hygiene. We felt that this would avoid "reinventing the wheel" but could potentially improve upon the existing CBT-I package. Therefore, our first mindfulness treatment program was a combination of mindfulness meditation and behavior therapy for insomnia as separate treatment components. This first prototype of MBTI included six sessions delivered weekly with each session lasting between 90 and 120 minutes. The intervention was conducted in a group format with seven or eight participants per group. The first session consisted of an orientation and introduction to the principles of mindfulness meditation including a few brief meditations. Sessions 2 through 5 consisted of mindfulness components and behavioral components for insomnia delivered separately. The first half of the session opened with formal guided meditations (e.g., breathing meditation, body scan, walking meditation, eating meditation), followed by group discussion. The second half consisted of instructions for the behavioral components, including sleep restriction and stimulus control, delivered sequentially across sessions. In addition to the sessions, participants were instructed to practice the meditation for at least 30 minutes per day, 5 days per week.

In our first study (Ong, Shapiro, & Manber, 2008), we enrolled 30 participants, 27 of whom completed the intervention. Because this study was designed as a proof-of-concept, there was no control group; at this stage of treatment development our aim was to see if our concept was feasible and acceptable. Overall, we found several significant pre- to posttreatment changes indicating that our intervention was making a positive impact on sleep parameters, thoughts about sleep, and sleep-related arousal (see Table 9.1). In addition, we examined several measures of clinical significance to determine if these changes were meaningful in a clinical context. Using the quantitative criteria for insomnia (Lichstein, Durrence, Taylor, Bush, & Riedel, 2003), defined as a sleep onset latency (SOL) greater than 30 minutes or wake after sleep onset (WASO) greater than 30 minutes at least three times per week, 87% of the sample no longer satisfied the criteria for insomnia at the end of treatment. Using a reduction of 50% or greater from baseline on total wake time (TWT) as an index of clinical significance, 50% of the participants in the sample met this criterion at the end of treatment. The average reduction was about 54 minutes of TWT from baseline. Finally, using validated cutoff scores on the Insomnia Severity Index (Bastien, Vallières, & Morin, 2001), 71% of the sample no longer met criteria for clinically significant insomnia at posttreatment. It is interesting to note that there was very little change in total sleep time (TST) from pre- to posttreatment. Although this might seem counterintuitive, studies on CBT-I often do not have significant increases in TST at posttreatment. This appears to be due to the reduction in time in bed that is part of the sleep restriction component, which was also used in this version of MBTI.

We also conducted a naturalistic follow-up on these participants at 6 and 12 months posttreatment to gather data on the long-term effects of the prototype MBTI (Ong et al., 2009). Using available data from 21 participants, we found that most benefits were maintained during the 12-month follow-up period. One noteworthy finding involved the relationship between sleep-related arousal and future episodes of insomnia. Participants who reported at least one insomnia episode during the follow-up period (defined as having 4 consecutive weeks with SOL >30 minutes or WASO >30 minutes at least three times each week) had significantly higher scores at posttreatment compared with those with no insomnia episodes on the Pre-Sleep Arousal Scale (Nicassio, Mendlowitz, Fussell, & Petras, 1985) and the Glasgow Sleep Effort Scale (Broomfield & Espie, 2005). This finding suggests that when sleep effort and presleep arousal remained elevated at the end of treatment, it constituted a higher risk for future occurrence of insomnia episodes during the follow-up period. Furthermore, since the data collected for episodes of insomnia occurred after participants completed the intervention, the temporal relationship of the data indicates that arousal and sleep effort precede the occurrence of insomnia rather than occur concurrently with insomnia. This would be consistent with the hypothesis that arousal is a risk factor as opposed to an epiphenomenon of sleep disturbance.

TABLE 9.1

Pretreatment to Posttreatment Changes

Measure	Pretreatment M	SD	Posttreatment M	SD	df	t	P	d
Sleep								
TWT (min)	107.91	60.68	53.47	41.61	29	6.39	<.001*	−1.17
SOL	39.09	35.47	20.82	22.06	29	4.58	<.001	−0.84
WASO	43.95	42.75	19.11	24.72	29	3.38	.002	−0.62
EMA	24.87	20.73	13.54	15.92	29	3.17	.004	−0.58
TST (min)	377.23	62.36	372.51	62.20	29	0.60	.553	−0.11
TIB (min)	484.45	72.14	425.40	56.14	29	5.32	<.001*	−0.97
SE (%)	78.54	10.57	87.62	9.75	29	6.20	<.001*	1.13
NWAK	2.21	1.79	1.22	1.35	27	3.35	.002*	−0.61
SQ	5.73	1.32	6.12	1.37	27	2.38	.025	0.45
Presleep arousal								
Total	34.73	8.94	28.03	9.02	29	5.48	<.001*	−1.00
Cognitive	21.10	6.05	16.47	6.06	29	5.20	<.001	−0.95
Somatic	13.63	4.33	11.57	4.26	29	3.78	.001	−0.69
Secondary measures								
Insomnia Severity Index	14.90	4.72	9.57	5.41	28	7.09	<.001*	−1.32
Dysfunctional Beliefs and Attitudes About Sleep	113.27	31.79	84.93	40.49	29	5.77	<.001*	−1.05
Hyperarousal Scale	66.50	10.00	63.83	8.93	29	2.53	.017	−0.46
Kentucky Inventory of Mindfulness Skills	129.93	11.78	131.83	16.19	29	0.97	.340	0.18
Glasgow Sleep Effort Scale	6.72	2.97	3.66	2.70	28	5.19	<.001*	−0.96
Positive and Negative Affect Schedule (Positive)	31.53	6.46	32.80	6.77	29	0.99	.328	0.18
Positive and Negative Affect Schedule (Negative)	18.30	5.76	16.77	5.20	29	2.00	.055	−0.37
Daytime Sleepiness	3.88	1.93	3.80	1.96	27	.263	.795	−.050
Daytime Tiredness	4.10	1.58	4.16	1.86	27	.296	.770	.050

Note. Sleep quality ranges from 1 (*very poor*) to 10 (*excellent*). Daytime sleepiness and tiredness are rated from 1 to 10, with higher numbers reflecting higher levels of sleepiness or tiredness, respectively. For Cohen's *d*, a positive value indicates an increase from pre- to posttreatment while a negative value indicates a decrease from pre- to posttreatment. TWT = total wake time; SOL = sleep onset latency; WASO = wake time after sleep onset; EMA = early morning awakenings; TST = total sleep time; TIB = time in bed; SE = sleep efficiency; NWAK = number of awakenings; SQ = sleep quality. From "Combining Mindfulness Meditation With Cognitive–Behavior Therapy for Insomnia: A Treatment-Development Study," by J. C. Ong, S. L. Shapiro, and R. Manber, 2008, *Behavior Therapy, 39,* p. 178. Copyright 2008 by Elsevier. Reprinted with permission.
*p < .05, with Bonferroni adjustment for multiple comparisons.

We also found several patterns consistent with the hypothesis that greater levels of mindfulness are associated with lower levels of daytime sleepiness and fatigue. Negative correlations (i.e., inverse relationship) were found between mindfulness skills, as measured by the Kentucky Inventory of Mindfulness Skills (Baer, Smith, & Allen, 2004), and self-reported daytime sleepiness. Also, a significant decrease in daytime fatigue was found from baseline to 6-month follow-up. There was a significant decrease in self-reported daytime fatigue at 6 months with only a modest 8-minute increase in TST during that same time frame, indicating that increased sleep time alone was unlikely to account for the improvement in daytime fatigue. These findings support the hypothesis that acquiring mindfulness skills might help improve waking functioning, specifically with reducing daytime sleepiness and fatigue.

LESSONS LEARNED

As a proof-of-concept, the first set of studies provided the necessary pilot data on feasibility, acceptability, and preliminary treatment effects to merit further testing of mindfulness meditation as an intervention for insomnia. In addition to the quantitative data described above, there were several lessons that we learned by gathering qualitative data from participants about their experience (Ong, Shapiro, & Manber, 2008). First, participants expressed overall satisfaction with the intervention, but they also expressed a desire to receive more meditations. They wanted to have more guidance on the meditation exercises during the sessions, and wanted to have a better conceptual understanding of how mindfulness meditation could improve sleep through anecdotes or case examples. As the clinician delivering the intervention, I observed a "tension" between maintaining a mindful position during the meditations and then having a more authoritative role in delivering instructions for sleep restriction or stimulus control. It felt awkward to encourage people to be mindful and explore during the first part of the session and then switch gears to instruct them on when to go to bed and when to get out of bed during the second part of the session. Also, my training as a clinical psychologist was primarily oriented in cognitive behavioral paradigms and I was relatively new to mindfulness, so I had limited experience in teaching mindfulness principles and leading meditations. As is typically done during the early phases of treatment development, we went back to the drawing board and worked on integrating the concepts of mindfulness meditation and behavior therapy to be more consistent and better integrated.

In revising the treatment package, we decided to shift from our original idea of adding mindfulness as a component of a behavioral treatment package, to delivering the components of behavior therapy for insomnia (sleep restriction, stimulus control, sleep hygiene), within the framework of a mindfulness-based intervention. We looked at how awareness from the mindfulness meditations could fit with the concepts from sleep physiology and behavior therapy that were being taught in the traditional delivery of sleep restriction and stimulus control. This led us to the notion that awareness of physical and mental states is important to know how and when to follow the instructions for sleep restriction and stimulus control. We also gave these terms a "facelift" and called them *sleep consolidation* and *sleep reconditioning*, respectively. This stemmed from the observation that participants found the term *sleep restriction* to imply something punitive and that *stimulus control* seemed to be a technical term that did not help participants understand the concept of the instructions. The end result was quite different from what we had originally set out to do. Rather than adding mindfulness meditation as another component of a multicomponent behavior therapy for insomnia, the behavior techniques were now woven into the framework of a mindfulness-based intervention. This gave rise to MBTI in its current form as an integrated, mindfulness-based intervention using the principles and practices of mindfulness meditation as the foundation for making metacognitive shifts in the context of insomnia.

TESTING EFFICACY: CONDUCTING A RANDOMIZED CONTROLLED TRIAL ON MBTI

Although our pilot studies were useful to determine the feasibility and acceptability of delivering mindfulness meditation for people with chronic insomnia, the study design did not allow us to draw conclusions regarding efficacy (i.e., whether or not the treatment works under controlled conditions). Determining the efficacy of MBTI requires a randomized controlled trial (RCT), a more sophisticated study that would entail greater costs. Using the pilot studies as preliminary data, we were fortunate to receive a research grant to support this next step in testing MBTI from the National Center for Complementary and Integrative Health (formerly known as the National Center for Complementary and Alternative Medicine), an institute within the National Institutes of Health.

There are many considerations that go into designing an RCT. After considering different options and receiving feedback from grant reviewers, we settled on a three-arm design that included MBTI, mindfulness-based stress reduction (MBSR), and a control condition with an 8-week self-monitoring period followed by an 8-week multicomponent behavior therapy for insomnia that did not include a cognitive component. This study was designed as a small-scale trial to generate initial evidence on efficacy. Definitive trials require very large sample sizes, a group of well-trained treatment providers to deliver the interventions, and efforts to ensure blinding wherever possible. These efforts require substantial resources that were beyond our capabilities at this stage of our research program. As we followed the stages of treatment development for behavior therapies (Rounsaville, Carroll, & Onken, 2001), the findings from this efficacy study were meant to inform the need for a more definitive large-scale study. Second, the decision to include both MBTI and MBSR as arms in this study was driven by the limitation of our pilot study (Ong, Shapiro, & Manber, 2008) that included both mindfulness and behavior therapy for insomnia, making it unclear how important mindfulness meditation was relative to the behavioral components. By including MBSR, widely recognized as the standard mindfulness meditation program, and comparing it with both MBTI and the control condition, we were able to generate evidence on the benefits of mindfulness meditation delivered alone (MBSR) and integrated with behavior therapy (MBTI). The control condition was designed to control for the effects of self-monitoring using sleep diaries as a parallel arm. Self-monitoring using sleep diaries has been shown to have mild effects on reducing SOL (Espie, Inglis, Tessier, & Harvey, 2001; Espie et al., 2012) and moderate effects on increasing sleep efficiency (Espie et al., 2012). Because all three arms would be completing daily sleep diaries during the 8-week treatment/monitoring period, controlling for self-monitoring would rule out the alternative hypothesis that changes in TWT derived from the sleep diaries were due to completing daily sleep diaries rather than the mindfulness interventions. Third, the theoretical framework of using mindfulness meditation is to target sleep-related arousal in the context of insomnia (see Chapter 4). Therefore, we selected individuals with a chronic insomnia disorder who also reported heightened arousal or anxiety about sleep. In previous versions of the *International Classification of Sleep Disorders* (*ICSD*; American Academy of Sleep Medicine, 2005), this was classified as psychophysiological insomnia. The third edition of the *ICSD* (American Academy of Sleep Medicine, 2014) now classifies this as a subtype of chronic insomnia disorder. Similarly, the fifth edition of the *Diagnostic and Statistical Manual of Mental Disorders* (American Psychiatric Association, 2013) classifies this as an insomnia disorder and does not distinguish subtypes.

The main outcome from our study was published in the journal *Sleep* (Ong et al., 2014). We randomized 54 participants with chronic insomnia to receive MBSR ($n = 19$), MBTI ($n = 19$), or self-monitoring ($n = 16$). The primary outcome measures were the Pre-Sleep Arousal Scale (PSAS; Nicassio, Mendlowitz, Fussell, & Petras, 1985) and TWT derived from sleep diaries. *Clinical significance* was defined as those who met criteria for treatment remission and treatment response using the Insomnia Severity Index (Bastien, Vallières, & Morin, 2001). The data analysis plan addressed two research questions. First, is mindfulness meditation delivered using MBSR, a standard meditation program, or delivered using MBTI, a tailored meditation program with behavior strategies for insomnia, superior to a self-monitoring (SM) control? Second, are there relative benefits for the tailored approach (MBTI) compared with the standard approach (MBSR) of delivering a meditation-based therapy?

The findings revealed that those receiving a mindfulness-based intervention (either MBSR or MBTI) had significantly greater reductions on TWT (43.75 minutes vs. 1.09 minutes), PSAS (7.13 vs. 0.16), and ISI (4.56 vs. 0.06) from baseline-to-post compared with SM (see Figure 9.1). Post hoc analyses revealed that MBSR and MBTI were each superior compared with SM on TWT, PSAS, and ISI, but no significant differences were found when comparing MBSR and MBTI with each other from baseline-to-post. However, significant differences emerged when the assessment timeframe included baseline to the 6-month follow-up. In these analyses, MBTI had greater reductions in ISI scores compared with MBSR, with the largest difference occurring at the 3-month follow-up. In terms of clinical significance, remission rates in the MBSR group were largely stable over time, (46.2% at post, 38.5% at 3 months, and 41.7% at 6 months), whereas remission rates for MBTI increased

FIGURE 9.1

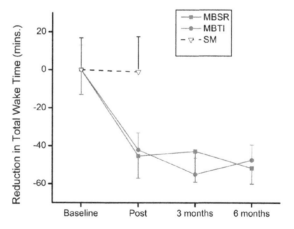

Change in total wake time. Total wake time (in minutes, with standard error of the mean) across study arms as reported in sleep diaries. Data presented are change scores from baseline to each assessment point. MBSR = mindfulness-based stress reduction; MBTI = mindfulness-based therapy for insomnia; SM = self-monitoring. From "A Randomized Controlled Trial of Mindfulness Meditation for Chronic Insomnia," by J. C. Ong, R. Manber, Z. Segal, Y. Xia, S. Shapiro, and J. K. Wyatt, 2014, *Sleep*, *37*, p. 1557. Copyright 2014 by Associated Professional Sleep Societies. Adapted with permission.

steadily from 33.3% at post to 38.5% at 3-month follow-up and 50% at 6-month follow-up (see Figure 9.2). Similarly, treatment response remained relatively steady between post and follow-up in MBSR (38.5% and 41.7%) but showed a steady increase from post (60%), 3-month (71.4%), and 6-month follow-up (78.6%) in MBTI.

In addition to these self-reported outcomes, polysomnography (PSG) and wrist actigraphy data were collected as objective measures of sleep. None of the PSG-measured sleep parameters were significantly different between the groups, although the patterns on TWT and TST were consistent with the directions observed in the sleep diary data. For actigraphy, the analyses revealed that the pooled meditation arms showed significantly greater rates of reduction in TWT (17.97 minutes) relative to SM. However, no significant differences between the groups were found at posttreatment. A similar finding was observed for TST, in which the meditation arms showed significantly greater rates of reduction in TST

FIGURE 9.2

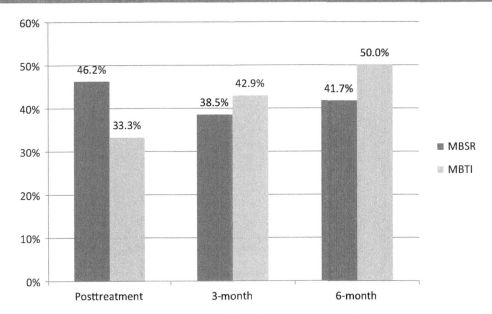

Treatment remission. Percentage of patients who met criteria for treatment remission defined as Insomnia Severity Index total score < 8 at each assessment point. Treatment remission for self-monitoring at posttreatment was 6.3% (not pictured). MBSR = mindfulness-based stress reduction; MBTI = mindfulness-based treatment for insomnia. From "A Randomized Controlled Trial of Mindfulness Meditation for Chronic Insomnia," by J. C. Ong, R. Manber, Z. Segal, Y. Xia, S. Shapiro, and J. K. Wyatt, 2014, Sleep, 37, p. 1559. Copyright 2014 by Associated Professional Sleep Societies. Adapted with permission.

compared with SM, but no significant differences between the groups were found at posttreatment. Although we did not find support for our hypotheses on these objective measures of sleep, it should be noted that these measures typically have smaller effects compared to self-reported measures. Two previous studies on mindfulness-based treatments found only small effect sizes on objective measures of sleep (Britton, Haynes, Fridel, & Bootzin, 2010; Gross et al., 2011). Overall, it appears that mindfulness meditation has larger effects on patient-reported sleep outcomes relative to objectively-measured sleep outcomes.

Data on treatment-process measures showed that participants had generally good adherence and attendance. The average attendance for all randomized participants was not significantly different between MBSR and MBTI, with the mean attendance of MBSR at 4.95 sessions and the mean attendance of MBTI at 5.74 sessions. Using six out of eight sessions as our "minimal therapeutic dose" for mindfulness, 12 out of the 16 participants who received MBSR attended at least six sessions and 11 out of the 18 participants who received MBTI attended at least six sessions. The majority of absences were due to scheduling conflicts or unexpected emergencies, and whenever possible instructors would review the content of the missed session and homework assignments over the phone at an alternate time. If the participant failed to attend without prior notice, the instructor would attempt to contact the participant and review the session materials and homework assignments to keep the participant engaged and maintain program continuity. A treatment credibility and expectancy questionnaire (Devilly & Borkovec, 2000) was completed by participants after Session 1 and prior to Session 3 so that they could provide ratings after having some initial exposure to the treatment condition. No significant differences were found between treatment conditions on credibility (logicalness, success in reducing symptoms, or confidence in recommending to friend) or expectancy (degree of expected improvement from treatment). With regard to meditation practice, data from the meditation diaries revealed that participants in MBSR averaged nearly 2,000 minutes of meditation practice during the study period, and participants in MBTI averaged a little under 1,300 minutes of meditation practice. MBSR participants reported significantly more home meditation sessions and more total minutes of home meditation practice compared to participants in MBTI. This should not be surprising since the recommendations for home meditation practice in MBTI is shorter (30 minutes) than MBSR (45 minutes). Finally, no treatment-related adverse events were reported, so mindfulness meditation appears to be safe for people with insomnia.

The overall conclusion from this study is that interventions using mindfulness meditation (either MBSR or MBTI) appear to be viable treatment options for people with chronic insomnia. Both MBSR and MBTI were superior to the self-monitoring control for reducing presleep arousal and TWT, our main outcome measures. In terms of clinical significance, the rates of remission and response found for both MBSR and MBTI are within a range that is comparable to that of other studies using CBT-I (Irwin, Cole, & Nicassio, 2006; Smith et al., 2002). MBTI had a somewhat more favorable long-term profile, with remission rates reaching 50% and a response rate of 78.6% at the 6-month follow-up. The finding of improvements in the follow-up period is consistent with conclusions drawn from a review and meta-analysis conducted on meditation (Goyal et al., 2014) and provides evidence of the long-term benefits of mindfulness meditation. Furthermore, this treatment approach appears to be safe, as no treatment-related adverse events were reported.

As mentioned earlier, this study was meant to be an initial test of efficacy, and questions remain that need to be addressed or taken into account when interpreting these findings. First, this sample was relatively small and consisted of 74% women, with about two thirds identifying their ethnic–racial demographic as non-Hispanic Caucasian. This raises questions about who is likely to seek out mindfulness-based treatments and whether men and other minority ethnic groups would achieve the same benefits as those found in our study sample. Interestingly, Caucasian women with a high level of education are a prominent demographic group that uses complementary and alternative medicine (Pearson, Johnson, & Nahin, 2006). Women are also at greater risk than men for insomnia (Zhang & Wing, 2006). In a separate study examining baseline data gathered as part of our recruitment for this study, we found gender differences in cognitive–emotional factors that are related to hyperarousal (Hantsoo, Khou, White, & Ong, 2013). Among women, negative emotions were most closely associated with elevated presleep arousal; whereas among men, an internal sleep locus of control was most closely associated with elevated presleep arousal. These differences in gender profile suggest that an intervention such as mindfulness meditation that targets emotion regulation might be a better fit to reduce presleep arousal in women. For men, more traditional cognitive techniques, such as cognitive restructuring or behavioral experiments that target the sleep locus of control, might be a better fit to reduce presleep arousal. Further research is needed to examine these potential moderators of treatment outcome for mindfulness meditation, which could help identify who is most likely to achieve benefits from MBTI.

Another limitation of the study is the number of providers available. Ideally, in an RCT, there is a group of providers who receive standardized training to deliver the study treatments, have similar levels of experience, and are blind to the study hypotheses and main outcome measures. As mentioned earlier, the limited resources available for this study precluded this possibility, and the approach that was taken was to select the best available therapist for each treatment arm. In the study, the MBSR instructors were all experienced, doctoral-level MBSR teachers, one of whom was a medical doctor and the other a clinical psychologist. Neither of these providers had any formal training in sleep medicine, and they were instructed to deliver MBSR as they normally would with no special attention given to sleep or insomnia. I served as the instructor for all MBTI groups, as I have training in behavioral sleep medicine, MBSR, and experience with the development of MBTI. Therefore, I am very familiar with this patient population and the concepts of insomnia. Given these differences, it is possible that investigator bias, treatment allegiance, or therapist skill level were plausible explanations for the observed differences between treatment arms.

Other Mindfulness- and Acceptance-Based Approaches to Treating Insomnia

MBTI is one approach for using mindfulness meditation to help people with insomnia. Beyond MBTI, there is a growing literature examining the use of mindfulness meditation or mindfulness principles, acceptance and commitment therapy (ACT), or a combination of these approaches with more traditional behavioral approaches for insomnia. There are now several RCTs on mindfulness-based interventions for insomnia and significant sleep disturbances (see Table 9.2). One RCT compared MBSR with eszopiclone for individuals with chronic insomnia (Gross et al., 2011). Significant improvements were found from baseline to posttreatment in both groups on a number of sleep parameters. Within the MBSR group, significant improvements were found on actigraphy-measured SOL and diary-measured SOL, TST, and sleep efficiency. This study was a small-scale trial with only 30 participants total (MBSR = 20, eszopiclone = 10) and thus was not sufficiently powered for between-group comparisons. Qualitative data collected from focus groups conducted on those who were in the MBSR arm of this trial revealed several positive benefits of mindfulness that included more global health benefits beyond the symptoms of insomnia (Hubbling, Reilly-Spong, Kreitzer, & Gross, 2014). Participants commented that although sleep time might not have increased, they were sleeping better, felt that they were waking up more refreshed, and felt less distressed about insomnia and were better able to cope when it occurred. These findings provide encouraging evidence to support the positive impact that MBSR can have on other territories of insomnia.

Black, O'Reilly, Olmstead, Breen, and Irwin (2015) conducted an RCT on adults ages 55 and older with moderate sleep disturbances, defined as a score greater than 5 on the Pittsburgh Sleep Quality Index

TABLE 9.2

Summary of Mindfulness-Based Therapies for Improving Sleep

Reference	Patient sample	Intervention	Intervention details	Sleep/insomnia outcome measure	Sleep/insomnia findings
Shapiro et al. (2003)	63 cancer-free women with previous diagnosis of Stage II breast cancer	Mindfulness-based stress reduction (MBSR)	Randomized to MBSR or free-choice control condition	Sleep efficiency and sleep quality measured by sleep diary	Both groups reported significant improvement in self-reported sleep quality at posttreatment; no significant change in sleep efficiency. MBSR participants reporting greater mindfulness practice showed largest improvement in sleep quality.
Andersen et al. (2013)	336 women undergoing surgery for Stage I–III breast cancer within the last 3–18 months	MBSR	Randomized to MBSR or treatment as usual control condition	Medical Outcomes Study Sleep Scale	Mean sleep problem scores were significantly lower in MBSR group immediately after the intervention but no lower than controls at 12-month follow-up.
Lengacher et al. (2012)	84 women who had completed breast cancer treatment within the last 18 months	MBSR	Randomized to 6-week MBSR intervention or treatment as usual control condition	M.D. Anderson Symptom Inventory core symptom severity items: Sleep disturbance, fatigue	MBSR group showed significant decrease in fatigue and sleep disturbance severity items at posttreatment compared to control group.
Carlson et al. (2003)	49 breast cancer and 10 prostate cancer patients	MBSR	Participants completed 8-week MBSR program	Self-reported sleep quality (poor, adequate, or good)	Significant improvement in sleep quality reported at posttreatment.

Study	Sample	Treatment	Design	Measure	Results
Carlson & Garland (2005)	63 cancer patients	MBSR	Participants completed 8-week MBSR program	Pittsburgh Sleep Quality Index (PSQI)	Significant improvement in PSQI total score and all PSQI subscales at posttreatment.
Schmidt et al. (2011)	177 women with fibromyalgia	MBSR	Randomized to MBSR, active control, or wait-list control	PSQI	No significant main effect for group; however, positive change rates on PSQI were highest for MBSR.
Gross et al. (2004)	20 solid organ transplant recipients	MBSR	Participants completed 8-week MBSR program	PSQI	Significant improvement in sleep dysfunction at post-treatment and 3-month follow-up.
Gross et al. (2010)	138 recipients of kidney, kidney/pancreas, liver, heart, or lung transplant	MBSR	Randomized to MBSR or 8-week health education intervention, either initially or after wait-list	PSQI	MBSR group reported significant improvement in sleep symptoms compared to Health Education; benefits were retained at 1-year follow-up.
Kreitzer et al. (2005)	20 solid organ transplant recipients	MBSR	Participants completed 8-week MBSR program	Self-reported sleep quality and duration	Significant improvements in sleep quality and duration sustained 6 months later.
Bootzin & Stevens (2005)	55 adolescents with substance abuse, insomnia, and daytime sleepiness	MBSR	Six-session group treatment for sleep disturbance combining MBSR, sleep hygiene education, and cognitive therapy	Sleep diary parameters (sleep efficiency, sleep onset latency, number of awakenings), Epworth Sleepiness Scale, actigraphy	Participants in MBSR group completing four or more treatment sessions reported significant improvement in sleep diary parameters; actigraphy showed a trend for improvement in total sleep. All participants reported significant reduction in sleepiness.
Klatt et al. (2009)	48 healthy university faculty and staff working full-time	Low-dose MBSR (MBSR-ld)	Randomized to 6-week MBSR-ld intervention or wait-list control	PSQI	Both MBSR-ld group and control group reported significant improvement in sleep quality at posttreatment.

(continues)

TABLE 9.2 (*Continued*)

Summary of Mindfulness-Based Therapies for Improving Sleep

Reference	Patient sample	Intervention	Intervention details	Sleep/insomnia outcome measure	Sleep/insomnia findings
Carmody et al. (2011)	110 late peri-menopausal and early post-menopausal women	MBSR	Randomized to MBSR or wait-list control	Women's Health Initiative Insomnia Rating Scale	MBSR group reported significantly greater improvements in subjective sleep quality compared with control group.
Garland et al. (2014)	111 cancer patients with insomnia	MBSR	Randomized to MBSR or eight sessions of cognitive behavior therapy for insomnia (CBT-I)	Insomnia Severity Index (ISI), PSQI, Dysfunctional Attitudes and Beliefs about Sleep Scale (DBAS), sleep diary parameters (sleep onset latency, wake time after sleep onset, total sleep time), actigraphy	MBSR was inferior to CBT-I for improving insomnia severity immediately post-intervention but demonstrated non-inferiority at 3-month follow-up. Both interventions showed improvement in sleep diary parameters. CBT-I group reported significant improvement in sleep quality and dysfunctional sleep beliefs.
Gross et al. (2011)	30 adults with primary chronic insomnia	MBSR	Randomized to MBSR or 8 weeks of pharmaco-therapy (3 mg of eszopiclone)	ISI, PSQI, sleep diary parameters (total sleep time, sleep onset latency, sleep efficiency), actigraphy	MBSR group reported significant improvements in insomnia severity, sleep quality, and sleep diary parameters at 5-month follow-up; comparable changes were seen in pharmacotherapy group. Actigraphy showed significant reductions in sleep onset latency for MBSR group.

Study	Sample	Intervention	Design	Measures	Results
Hubbling et al. (2014)	18 adults with chronic insomnia	MBSR	Randomized to MBSR	Qualitative data collected via posttreatment focus groups	Participants receiving MBSR reported improved sleep quality and reduced insomnia-related distress.
Britton et al. (2010)	26 adults with partially remitted depression	Mindfulness-based cognitive therapy (MBCT)	Randomized to MBCT or wait-list control	Polysomnographic (PSG) sleep profiles, sleep diary parameters (sleep onset latency, number of awakenings, wake time after sleep onset, sleep efficiency)	Polysomnography showed increased arousal at posttreatment in MBCT group (increased awakenings, Stage 1 sleep, suppressed slow wave sleep). MBCT group reported significant within-group decreases in sleep diary parameters.
Britton et al. (2012)	23 antidepressant users with sleep complaints	MBCT	Randomized to MBCT or wait-list control	PSG (Stage 1 sleep, slow-wave sleep), sleep diary parameters (total wake time, sleep efficiency)	MBCT group showed a significant reduction in PSG total wake time and significant improvement in sleep diary parameters.
Yook et al. (2008)	19 patients with anxiety disorders	MBCT	Participants completed 8 weeks of MBCT	PSQI	Participants showed significant improvement in sleep quality at posttreatment.
Gonzalez-Garcia et al. (2013)	40 adults diagnosed with HIV	MBCT	Randomized to MBCT intervention or routine follow-up control	Nottingham Health Profile–Sleep dimension score	MBCT group showed significant improvement in sleep-related quality of life at Week 8 and Week 20.
Heidenreich et al. (2006)	14 adults with persistent primary insomnia	MBCT	Participants completed MBCT	Sleep diary parameters (sleep latency, total sleep time), Questionnaire to Assess Central Personality Variables in Insomnia, Thoughts Control Questionnaire for insomnia (TCQ-I)	Participants showed significant pre- to posttreatment improvements in sleep diary parameters; fewer participants were taking sleep medications at end of treatment. Significant changes were seen across treatment in four of six subscales of the TCQ-I; patients reported significantly less worry about sleep.

(continues)

TABLE 9.2 (Continued)

Summary of Mindfulness-Based Therapies for Improving Sleep

Reference	Patient sample	Intervention	Intervention details	Sleep/insomnia outcome measure	Sleep/insomnia findings
Ong et al. (2008)	30 adults with psychophysiological insomnia	Mindfulness-based therapy for insomnia (MBTI)	6-week multi-component intervention incorporating mindfulness meditation and CBT-I	Sleep diary parameters (total wake time, time in bed, number of awakenings), ISI, Hyperarousal Scale, DBAS, Glasgow Sleep Effort Scale (GSES), Pre-sleep Arousal Scale (PSAS)	Participants reported significant posttreatment improvements in sleep diary parameters, insomnia severity, presleep arousal, sleep effort, and dysfunctional sleep-related cognitions.
Ong et al. (2014)	54 adults with chronic insomnia	MBSR, MBTI	Randomized to MBSR, MBTI, or 8-week self-monitoring condition	Total wake time measured by sleep diary, ISI, Pre-Sleep Arousal Scale (PSAS), PSG, actigraphy	MBTI and MBSR were associated with significantly greater reductions in total wake time, presleep arousal, and insomnia severity compared to controls. MBTI group had greater reductions in ISI scores compared with MBSR.
Black et al. (2015)	49 older adults with moderate sleep disturbances	Mindful Awareness Practices (MAPs)	Randomized to 6-week MAPs or Sleep Hygiene Education (SHE) intervention	Pittsburgh Sleep Quality Index (PSQI), Athens Insomnia Scale (AIS), Fatigue Symptom Inventory (FSI)	Compared with SHE, MAPs group showed greater posttreatment improvements in PSQI scores, insomnia symptoms, and fatigue severity and interference.

Note. From "Third-Wave Therapies for Insomnia," by H. L. Taylor, H. P. Hailes, and J. Ong, 2015, *Current Sleep Medicine Reports, 1,* p. 173. Copyright 2015 by Springer. Adapted with permission.

(PSQI; Buysse, Reynolds, Monk, Berman, & Kupfer, 1989), that compared a 6-week mindfulness-based group intervention called mindfulness awareness practices (MAP) against a 6-week group consisting of sleep hygiene education that controlled for attention and contact. There was a significant group decrease in PSQI scores for the MAP group but not the sleep hygiene control group, and the change in PSQI was significantly correlated with the change in scores on the Five Facets of Mindfulness Scale (Baer, Smith, Hopkins, Krietemeyer, & Toney, 2006), indicating that increased mindfulness skills were associated with decreased symptoms of sleep disturbances among participants who received MAP. MAP was also superior to the sleep hygiene control on daytime measures of fatigue and the Beck Depression Inventory (Beck, Steer, & Carbin, 1988), thus indicating improvement in other domains related to sleep. Notably, 67% of the participants were women and 84% were White, with an average of 16.6 years of education. These demographics are similar to our study (Ong et al., 2014) and continue the trend of a demographic pattern in mindfulness-based treatment studies.

Several other studies have examined insomnia or sleep disturbances that are comorbid with another psychiatric or medical disorder. One of the most common co-occurring psychiatric disorders with insomnia is mood disorder. Britton has conducted two small-scale randomized controlled trials examining mindfulness-based cognitive therapy (MBCT) compared with a wait-list control for people with unipolar depression and insomnia. The first study (Britton et al., 2010) examined individuals with depression and comorbid insomnia who were not on medication. Participants in both groups reported reductions in SOL on sleep diaries, but data from polysomnography found that participants in the MBCT group had significantly more awakenings, increased Stage 1 sleep, and decreased slow-wave sleep relative to controls. The authors interpreted these findings as indices of cortical arousal that appear to mimic the effects typically found among antidepressant users. The second study (Britton, Haynes, Fridel, & Bootzin, 2012) examined individuals with depression and comorbid insomnia who were taking antidepressant medication. The results revealed that those who received MBCT had less TWT and higher sleep efficiencies compared with the control group on both objective (polysomnography) and self-report (sleep diaries) measures of sleep. Besides depression, there is evidence for improvements in self-reported sleep quality following MBCT for individuals suffering from insomnia related to an anxiety disorder (Yook et al., 2008). Another study using a multicomponent treatment that included mindfulness meditation found evidence for improvements in sleep and reductions in relapse of substance use among adolescents with a substance abuse history (Bootzin & Stevens, 2005).

Among comorbid medical conditions, particular interest has centered on the use of mindfulness-based approaches on cancer-related sleep disturbance and fatigue. One early study examined the impact of MBSR on self-reported sleep quality and quantity among women with breast cancer (Shapiro, Bootzin, Figueredo, Lopez, & Schwartz, 2003). No differences were found between the MBSR and the control group on sleep quality and sleep efficiency, but a positive relationship was found between the practice of mindfulness techniques and feeling refreshed after sleep for the MBSR group. In a series of studies, Carlson, Speca, Patel, and Goodey (2003) found evidence that MBSR leads to improvements in sleep quality among those with breast and prostate cancer and among a heterogeneous group of cancer patients (Carlson & Garland, 2005). Another study using a noninferiority design (Garland et al., 2014) compared MBSR with CBT-I in an RCT on patients with cancer. At posttreatment, MBSR was found to be inferior to CBT-I for improving insomnia severity but demonstrated noninferiority at the 3-month follow-up. At the final follow-up assessment, similar reductions in SOL and wake after sleep onset were found for both MBSR and CBT-I. These findings give rise to the possibility of different mechanisms to reduce insomnia severity, with CBT-I exerting direct effects on nocturnal symptoms and MBSR indirectly improving sleep by improving the quality of daytime functioning (e.g., reduction in mood disturbance, stress).

In addition to mindfulness-based therapies, there has been some work to date on using ACT for patients with insomnia. One case study (Dalrymple, Fiorentino, Politi, & Posner, 2010) reported on the successful treatment of an individual with insomnia using behavioral strategies with acceptance-based strategies. A pilot study examined the use of ACT for 11 patients with chronic insomnia who were nonresponders to traditional CBT-I (Hertenstein et al., 2014). They found that at posttreatment these patients reported improvements in sleep-related quality of life and sleep quality. These two studies provide some indication that acceptance-based treatments might provide benefits for people with insomnia, particularly those not responding to CBT-I. See Table 9.2 for a list of mindfulness-based treatment studies on sleep and insomnia.

Future Research Directions

These are exciting times for research using mindfulness and acceptance-based approaches for chronic insomnia. The literature has grown considerably over the past 10 years, with increasing evidence to support the efficacy of mindfulness meditation as a viable treatment for chronic insomnia. Although these are positive signs, there are still some key questions that remain to be answered.

One important issue related to efficacy is the use of subjective versus objective outcome measures. In the studies reviewed, the main outcomes are self-report measures, mostly using sleep diaries or a global measure of insomnia symptoms, such as the Insomnia Severity Index. Studies that used objective measures have found very little change in sleep parameters (Britton et al., 2010; Gross et al., 2011; Ong et al., 2014). The inconsistencies between subjective and objective measures of sleep raise questions about the potential for a response bias due to expectancy effects or demand characteristics. However, self-report measures using sleep diaries and global measures of insomnia symptoms are considered to be a valid index for evaluating efficacy in insomnia studies (Buysse, Ancoli-Israel, Edinger, Lichstein, & Morin, 2006). In the case of insomnia, the perception of sleep plays a role in the insomnia disorder that is not captured in objective measures of sleep. Perhaps one way to minimize the potential for a response bias is to use blinding in the assessment process. For example, the study assessments could include a clinician rating that is administered by a member of the research team who is unaware of the participant's randomized condition. Although this step would not eliminate the possibility of a response bias, collecting assessment data from multiple sources and employing techniques for blinding could at least illuminate the potential for a response bias.

Another key question relates to the treatment mechanisms underlying MBTI and other mindfulness-based therapies. How do these treatments work? In Chapter 4, the conceptual model for MBTI is presented, but we have not yet collected any evidence to support our model. Therefore, studies are needed to determine how best to measure metacognitions that are relevant for insomnia and also to examine whether mindfulness meditation does indeed produce changes in metacognitions. It is also possible that practicing mindfulness meditation will lead to changes in the brain. One potential area that has been proposed involves the default mode network (DMN). The DMN is a network of systems in the brain that regulates self-referential thought during inactive waking periods, such as daydreaming, that is associated with mind wandering. One review paper proposed the possibility that the DMN plays a role in insomnia (Marques, Gomes, Clemente, dos Santos, & Castelo-Branco, 2015). Earlier, I discussed theories related to how insomnia might involve an inability to dearouse, which would be consistent with a dysregulation in the DMN around bedtime. Further investigation into this area might unveil neural mechanisms underlying mindfulness and insomnia.

Finally, it remains to be seen whether the version of MBTI presented here is the optimal treatment package. In Chapter 8, I discussed other modules and activities that could be integrated into an MBTI program. These include the loving-kindness meditation and explicit discussions of emotion-focused coping and problem-focused coping. Also, having follow-up sessions beyond the 8-week program could be used to enhance the long-term effects of MBTI. As noted at the beginning of this chapter, treatment development is an iterative process of refinement, and testing these variants could help improve the impact of MBTI.

Beyond insomnia, it might be possible to examine the potential use of mindfulness meditation for other types of sleep disorders. We are currently working on a project to repurpose and modify the MBTI program for people with chronic hypersomnia, including narcolepsy and idiopathic hypersomnia. Individuals with chronic hypersomnia have a tremendous psychological burden, including a high prevalence of depression and anxiety that appears to be associated with the burden of coping with chronic sleepiness. Given the potential benefits of targeting metacognitions to reduce sleep-related distress and daytime fatigue, this project aims to teach those with hypersomnia, similar concepts related to relieving suffering by learning how to be present and mindful with their condition. Unlike MBTI, this treatment model is an integrative model, which would include the use of approved medications for people with chronic hypersomnia, such as stimulants and sodium oxybate. This serves as an example of the potential outreach of using mindfulness to help people with a variety of sleep disturbances.

Delivering MBTI in the Real World

10

P eople with chronic insomnia now have more treatment options. The emergence of mindfulness-based therapy for insomnia (MBTI) and other programs that use mindfulness meditation provide an integrative approach, a unique set of tools, and a different way to think about the problem of insomnia. If mindfulness-based approaches can be considered a viable treatment option, how do they fit into the existing landscape of treatments? Should MBTI be a first-line treatment, or should people with insomnia first try to use sleep medication or cognitive behavior therapy for insomnia (CBT-I)? Are insurance companies going to pay for their patients to receive MBTI? In this chapter, I provide my perspective on some issues and areas of controversy related to the implementation of MBTI into real-world health care systems. The chapter concludes with some resources for readers who wish to continue their journey into mindfulness meditation and behavioral sleep medicine.

http://dx.doi.org/10.1037/14952-011
Mindfulness-Based Therapy for Insomnia, by J. C. Ong

Patient Considerations

Which patients should consider using mindfulness meditation to help with their sleep problem? In Part I of this book, I distinguished insomnia as a disorder versus the nocturnal symptoms of sleep disturbance. As discussed in Chapter 4, our conceptual model (Ong, Ulmer, & Manber, 2012) posits that mindfulness skills can target sleep-related metacognitions that arise during an insomnia disorder. Furthermore, the majority of the activities in MBTI were designed for those who have been experiencing insomnia symptoms for a prolonged period of time because sleep-related arousal is a perpetuating factor of chronic insomnia. Therefore, MBTI is most appropriate for patients with a chronic insomnia disorder. However, other programs teaching mindfulness meditation might be suitable for those who experience significant sleep disturbances but do not yet meet the full criteria for an insomnia disorder. Recall in Chapter 9, the study by Black, O'Reilly, Olmstead, Breen, and Irwin (2015) used a 6-week program called mindfulness awareness practices (MAP) that targeted older adults with prodromal sleep disturbances. Therefore, it is possible that teaching mindfulness meditation can also help prevent the development of chronic insomnia for those who have symptoms of insomnia in the form of moderate sleep disturbances. Conceptually, this would still fit within the 3-P model (Spielman, Caruso, & Glovinsky, 1987), whereby mindfulness meditation would help to reduce the impact of the precipitating event that created the initial sleep disturbance and also reduce the perpetuating factors that maintain the sleep disturbances. Moreover, this provides flexibility in terms of the target audience for mindfulness-based programs, which is important because of the heterogeneity of insomnia patients.

Thus far, it appears that the majority of participants in the randomized controlled trials on mindfulness and insomnia are women. In the three largest randomized controlled trials (Black et al., 2015; Garland et al., 2014; Ong et al., 2014), two thirds to three quarters of participants were women, most were Caucasian, and the level of education was relatively high. Is it the case that women are more likely than men to be interested in an intervention using mindfulness meditation? Or is it the case the mindfulness meditation is a better treatment match for reducing sleep-related arousal, which seems to be more elevated in women than men? A more interesting question to consider is who is an appropriate candidate across different treatment modalities, such as MBTI, CBT-I, and medications. Further research that could identify ways to match patients to treatment modalities based on clinical profiles could greatly enhance efficiency within a health care system.

Another set of patient consideration involves the medical and psychiatric comorbidities and the concurrent use of hypnotic medications during MBTI. As is typical for an early stage of research focusing on efficacy, we have only tested MBTI on insomnia patients who did not have significant medical or psychiatric comorbidities and who were not using hypnotic medications. The rationale for these exclusionary criteria was based on scientific reasons for isolating the effects of mindfulness meditation and avoiding possible confounders. It was not based on clinical counterindications. Thus, we do not have empirical evidence to suggest whether MBTI is appropriate for those on hypnotic medications or whether those who have depression or chronic medical conditions would receive the same benefits. From my clinical experience, I feel that patients with chronic medical conditions, such as chronic pain or chronic obstructive pulmonary disease would not present a barrier to engaging in MBTI, as long as the medical condition is stable. As reviewed in Chapter 3, mindfulness-based stress reduction (MBSR) and other mindfulness-based programs have been successful in helping patients with chronic medical conditions.

For psychiatric conditions, my clinical experience is that those with anxiety disorders tend to do well with MBTI, and other mindfulness and acceptance-based programs have been successful in treating those with active anxiety disorders (Hoge et al., 2013; Orsillo, Roemer, Lerner, & Tull, 2004). On the other hand, those with mood disorders, especially those who are experiencing significant symptoms of depression, can be vulnerable to dropping out of the program and might not having the ability to properly engage in the treatment. In one of our earlier research studies (Ong, Kuo, & Manber, 2008), we found that elevated levels of depression (as defined by a score ≥16 on the Beck Depression Inventory [Beck, Rush, Shaw, & Emery, 1979]) was the second most common predictor of early dropout from a group-delivered CBT-I, behind an average total sleep time of less than 4 hours. Given the overlap between CBT-I and MBTI, the same issue might also apply to dropouts in MBTI. Also, the mindfulness-based cognitive therapy (MBCT) program typically requires patients to be in remission for depression rather than in an active state of depression because patients in an active state of depression often do not have the cognitive and physical resources to engage in MBCT (Segal, Williams, & Teasdale, 2002).

It is still unclear whether MBTI is appropriate for patients who are using hypnotic medications. On the one hand, mindfulness can be very helpful for patients to let go of the need to rely on medications and the anxiety that is created when trying to decide whether one should take a sleeping pill on a given night. On the other hand, patients using sleep medication while participating in MBTI might attribute the improvements to the medications rather than to the practice of mindfulness principles.

Given that there is no evidence yet to provide guidance one way or the other, a prudent approach might be to allow patients to participate in MBTI who are on a stable dose and who still experience symptoms of insomnia because the medication has not sufficiently resolved the insomnia symptoms. However, if patients are just beginning to take sleep medication, or if their sleep is improved with sleep medication, then it might make more sense to have them first monitor the impact of the medication on their insomnia symptoms before deciding whether MBTI is appropriate. An alternative would be to introduce some medication-tapering elements into MBTI. This would likely require some modification to MBTI but could be another way to use mindfulness principles to help people with insomnia. Before attempting to taper or change the patient's sleep medication, MBTI instructors should consult with the prescribing physician. Most physicians would prefer to have their patients eventually sleep without a hypnotic medication, but these decisions should be coordinated between the MBTI instructor and the patient's physician. These recommendations are based on my clinical experience; future research studies can aid in providing empirical answers to these questions.

A potentially controversial question is whether people with different demographic characteristics, such as those of lower socioeconomic status or those with lower education, are appropriate candidates for MBTI. Generally, the participants that we have recruited have at least a college degree, so the data for patients with lower levels of education are not available to empirically answer this question. Anecdotally, I would say that demographic factors such as socioeconomic status and level of education do not seem to distinguish participants who connect with the values of MBTI and who report benefits. In other areas, mindfulness meditation has been successfully delivered in programs to low-income, ethnic minority elementary school children (Black & Fernando, 2014) and incarcerated adults with substance abuse issues (Bowen et al., 2006). It seems that people across different ages, levels of education, and socioeconomic status can benefit from the practice of mindfulness meditation. Again, further research could help clarify this question.

One final patient consideration is the composition of the group with respect to the presenting complaint. When Kabat-Zinn developed MBSR, it was designed to be a general program where people with different issues could come together to work on the common theme of suffering and stress. However, the nature and source of the suffering and stress would vary from person to person. Some might be experiencing chronic pain, others might have been diagnosed with cancer, and others might have sleep problems. The variety in suffering was thought to enhance the group's understanding of how mindfulness is a general practice and not an antidote or medical treatment for a particular condition. In contrast, MBTI is specifically designed for people with insomnia so everyone coming to an MBTI group should be experiencing at least some form of sleep disturbance, or it would not be relevant to them. In one of our pilot groups, we had an experienced MBSR instructor lead an MBSR class for a group of 12 patients with insomnia. Around the midway point, I asked the instructor how the class was going and he commented that there was something that felt different. He noted that because all participants had chronic insomnia and he had never experienced prolonged bouts of insomnia, there seemed to be a disconnect between the participants and himself that was not apparent to him in previous MBSR classes in which the participants were more diverse with regard to presenting complaints. He felt that this led to a polarization between group members and himself, which was completely unexpected for both him and me. We have since attempted to increase the heterogeneity of our groups by trying to have a range of patients of different ages, backgrounds, and other demographic characteristics whenever possible. Other ways to increase heterogeneity might be to include those with comorbid insomnia or those who are taking sleep medication, as discussed earlier.

Provider Considerations

This book is meant to be a starting point for those who are interested in delivering MBTI or teaching mindfulness meditation as a means of reducing symptoms of insomnia. As I have stated throughout this book, my position is that those who are considering using mindfulness meditation in a medical or psychiatric practice or teaching MBTI as part of an educational setting should be committed to practicing the principles of mindfulness. This begins by having a personal meditation practice and embodying the principles of mindfulness as a way of living. Those who do not have any experience with meditation might start by taking an MBSR class (or similar mindfulness-based program) to gain firsthand experience as a participant. Those who have an established meditation practice should consider attending a meditation retreat, which allows one to deepen the connection with mindfulness principles while also connecting with a community of other meditation practitioners. Moving forward, it is recommended that MBTI instructors continue to reinforce their meditation practice with regular attendance at a meditation retreat or meditation group. While there is no minimum competency for meditation practice, these suggestions are designed to foster a commitment to practicing mindfulness principles and enable MBTI instructors to bring mindfulness into their work with patients.

The professional competency needed to deliver MBTI is an area that is potentially controversial. Recall from earlier chapters that MBTI should be delivered by clinicians with appropriate training in mental health and/ or medical services that meet the standards set forth by their respective professional organizations. This level of competency ensures that the MBTI instructor is capable of making clinical decisions regarding whether or not a patient is stable enough to engage in MBTI or handling medical or psychiatric issues that might arise during the course of MBTI. Given the overlap between insomnia and other psychiatric and medical comorbidities, there is a high likelihood that an MBTI instructor will encounter a medical or psychiatric issue. Thus, MBTI is best suited for licensed, doctoral-level clinicians, such as clinical psychologists or physicians who are familiar with behavioral medicine and have some experience working with patients who have sleep disorders. These clinicians would likely require additional training in teaching mindfulness meditation or training in working with insomnia patients. Master's-level providers, such as nurses, clinical social workers, psychologists, and licensed marriage and family therapists, can also deliver MBTI. However, they might require more training than doctoral-level providers or need more experience working with insomnia patients.

This level of competency might seem restrictive, as some MBSR instructors are not licensed clinicians and yet could still be very effective at delivering MBTI. Furthermore, some would argue that an established personal meditation practice should be the primary determinant of competency to deliver a mindfulness-based therapy. Although these are valid arguments, the potential risks of working with people who have insomnia warrant a conservative approach at this time. It is possible that changes in health care regulation could reclassify mindfulness-based therapies as an educational class under integrative medicine as opposed to a form of psychotherapy. Perhaps future research on health service and provider competency could open up opportunities to reevaluate this standard.

Although there are no formal certifications for delivering MBTI, there are certifications and formal training for instructors who wish to deliver other types of mindfulness-based therapies. The Center for Mindfulness at the University of Massachusetts offers certification as an MBSR teacher (see Exhibit 10.1). There are also several training opportunities for teaching MBCT, including online training and 5-day professional training institutes offered at the University of California, San Diego; University of Toronto; and Oxford University.

In addition to training on mindfulness, training in behavioral sleep medicine (BSM) is important in the delivery of MBTI. The American Board of Sleep Medicine offers a Certification in Behavioral Sleep Medicine that covers the broad practice of BSM. As noted earlier, the American Psychological Association (APA) recently approved sleep psychology as a recognized specialty, and efforts are underway to develop an examination and certification for sleep psychology under the American Board of Professional Psychology. Although not required to deliver MBTI, obtain-

EXHIBIT 10.1

Further Resources on Mindfulness and Insomnia

Online Resources for Additional Training in Mindfulness-Based Therapies or Sleep Medicine
Center for Mindfulness, Training Pathway for certification as an MBSR teacher: http://www.
  umassmed.edu/cfm/training/training-pathways/
Mindfulness-Based Cognitive Therapy (MBCT) Training: http://mbct.com/training/
Oxford Mindfulness Centre: http://www.oxfordmindfulness.org/
Society of Behavioral Sleep Medicine (SBSM): http://www.behavioralsleep.org/
American Academy of Sleep Medicine (AASM): http://www.aasmnet.org/

Meditation Retreat Centers
Spirit Rock (http://www.spiritrock.org): Meditation Center in Northern California (about
  45 minutes north of San Francisco)
Insight Meditation Society (http://www.dharma.org): Meditation Center in Barre, Massachusetts

Online Resources for Scientific Programs in Meditation or Sleep Research
Mind and Life Institute: https://www.mindandlife.org/
Sleep Research Society: http://www.sleepresearchsociety.org/

Recommended Books on Mindfulness and Mindfulness-Based Therapies
Kabat-Zinn, J. (1990). *Full catastrophe living: The program of the stress reduction clinic at the
  University of Massachusetts Medical Center.* New York, NY: Delta.
Kabat-Zinn, J. (1994). *Wherever you go, there you are: Mindfulness meditation in everyday
  life.* New York, NY: Hyperion Books.
Kabat-Zinn, J. (2005). *Coming to our senses: Healing ourselves and the world through mind-
  fulness.* New York, NY: Hachette Books.
Segal, Z. V., Williams, J. M. G., & Teasdale, J. D. (2012). *Mindfulness-based cognitive therapy
  for depression* (2nd ed.). New York, NY: Guilford Press.
Stahl, B., & Goldstein, E. (2010). *A mindfulness-based stress reduction workbook.* Oakland, CA:
  New Harbinger.

Recommended Books on Insomnia and Behavioral Sleep Medicine
Glovinsky, P., & Spielman, A. (2006). *The insomnia answer: A personalized program for identifying
  and overcoming the three types of insomnia.* New York, NY: Penguin.
Lichstein, K. L., & Perlis, M. L. (Eds.). (2003). *Treating sleep disorders: Principles and practice of
  behavioral sleep medicine.* Hoboken, NJ: Wiley.
Morin, C. M. (1993). *Insomnia: Psychological assessment and management.* New York, NY:
  Guilford Press.
Morin, C. M., & Espie, C. A. (Eds.). (2003). *Insomnia: A clinician's guide to assessment and
  treatment* (Vol. 1). Dordrecht, the Netherlands: Springer Science & Business Media.

---

ing one of these certifications would ensure a minimum level of knowledge in BSM. Related to these efforts, the Society of Behavioral Sleep
Medicine offers continuing education courses in BSM that are generally
aimed at physicians, nurses, and psychologists who are interested in
working with people who have sleep disorders. There are also workshops and postgraduate courses at the annual international conference for sleep medicine that is organized by the Associated Professional
Sleep Societies. These are all excellent training opportunities to increase
knowledge about BSM, including insomnia, sleep physiology, and sleep

assessment techniques. Those interested in delivering MBTI are highly encouraged to use these training opportunities to integrate knowledge about insomnia, sleep regulation, stress, and health with the principles of mindfulness meditation.

Other Considerations for Delivery of MBTI

In addition to considerations at the patient and provider levels, there are important considerations for delivering mindfulness-based therapies at a broader system level. Thus far, MBTI has only been delivered within the context of a research study at a sleep disorders center. Other mindfulness-based therapies have been delivered in hospitals but are offered through psychotherapy clinics or more general educational settings rather than a specialty clinic in sleep disorders. Most mindfulness-based therapies can be delivered in any setting, as long as there is sufficient space to hold movement meditation practices and to comfortably house a group of participants. Depending on who the patients are (i.e., all insomnia patients or a mixed group) and how they are recruited (e.g., from a sleep disorders center, general announcements and fliers in a hospital), the circumstances might dictate where the most appropriate location is to hold the class or program. If the patient population is specific (e.g., all insomnia patients), then there should be some connection to a sleep disorders clinic to provide resources for an overnight sleep study or further evaluation for other sleep disorders, if needed. Similarly, if the group includes those with medical conditions, access to a primary care clinic or some other medical support would be important.

At a broader system level, mindfulness-based therapies do not fit cleanly into a category within most health care systems, because they contain elements of an educational class, psychotherapy, and alternative medicine. Earlier, I made the case that MBTI should be considered an integrative approach with techniques that aim to reduce specific symptoms of insomnia integrated with techniques that aim to promote emotion regulation and general well-being. In the United States, integrative health interventions are widely used by consumers, but important issues pertaining to reimbursement of services (for both the practitioner and patient) and regulation of these interventions remain unresolved. Most insurance companies in the United States do not currently pay for their customers to attend a mindfulness-based therapy, such as MBSR, which can range between $400 and $600 per class. Therefore, patients have to pay out-of-pocket for these services. Some patients have been able to use money from a flexible spending account as part of their health insurance to pay for a mindfulness behavior therapy (MBT), if they are able to receive a letter of medical necessity from their health care provider. Unfortunately, these financial considerations might present barriers to those in a lower socioeconomic status who cannot afford to pay out of pocket or who do not have a flexible spending account established. Hopefully, health care reforms, such as the Affordable Care Act, will provide greater opportunity for everyone to have a fair chance to access mindfulness-based therapies.

Another issue related to delivery of MBTI in the health care system is that there is currently no formal regulation with regard to provider qualification or quality of care. Earlier, I provided a perspective on provider qualifications for delivering MBTI. However, there is currently no method of regulating whether or not MBTI or other MBTs are being delivered with fidelity to the original program, which can raise questions about the quality of care. Ideally, a responsible clinician will provide his or her patients with the opportunity to provide feedback or have a formal program evaluation that patients can complete anonymously. These can be useful tools to continue to improve as an MBTI provider. Also, if there are other MBT instructors in the local area, it might be helpful to consider forming a peer group consisting of MBT teachers. This could include providers of MBSR, MBCT, MBTI, or other MBTs, since many challenges will be relevant to the core teaching of mindfulness meditation. As an example, there is an MBSR/MBCT teachers' consortium in Chicago that meets monthly to engage in meditation practice, discuss issues that teachers are encountering in delivering MBTs, and provide peer-support for delivering MBTs. This has provided a very useful and meaningful outlet for teachers to share their experiences in teaching MBTs. This can also provide opportunities to standardize the quality of care across MBTs. Hopefully, the growing evidence base on mindfulness-based therapies will persuade policymakers to address the issues related to implementation of mindfulness into the health care system.

A Vision for the Future

There are now more empirically supported treatment options for individuals who suffer from insomnia. Pharmacological approaches are becoming safer and more targeted in their pharmacodynamics. The z-drugs, melatonin agonists, and more recent orexin antagonists are more specific when compared with the older generation of pharmacological approaches to insomnia, which included barbiturates and benzodiazepines. Similarly, advances in nonpharmacological approaches have increased the range of treatment targets to address different symptoms of insomnia. CBT-I is more comprehensive compared with the older generation of behavioral approaches, which included relaxation strategies, mental imagery, or paradoxical intention. MBTI expands the armamentarium of nonpharmacological approaches by providing tools grounded in mindfulness meditation to reduce sleep-related arousal by targeting metacognitions. It provides a different way to work with the problem of insomnia than do medications or CBT-I. Therefore, it might be time to consider a systems-based approach to the treatment of insomnia.

One such approach could be accomplished using a stepped care model. Most patients first report their sleep problems to their primary care physician. If reported early on, this would likely fall under the category of acute insomnia or sleep disturbances. Therefore, a reasonable starting point might be a short-term trial of a hypnotic medication and some education about behaviors that are incompatible with sleep (e.g., sleep hygiene). Alternatively, if there is a resource for a BSM provider (e.g., nurse practitioner, primary care psychologist) in the clinic or nearby, the patient could be referred for a brief behavioral treatment for insomnia, such as the one developed by Dr. Daniel Buysse and colleagues (Buysse et al., 2011). If the sleep disturbance persists and transforms from acute sleep disturbance to a chronic insomnia disorder, then a higher level of expertise might be required as the patient moves up the stepped care model. Here, the patient might be referred to a sleep center for evaluation of comorbid sleep disorders and more specific information on the symptom patterns. If the patient reports increased sleep-related arousal and is open to a mindfulness-based approach, then the patient can be referred to an MBTI program. Alternatively, if the evaluation reveals a pattern of distorted cognitions or maladaptive behaviors, then the patient might benefit from a full course of CBT-I. If the patient continues to experience persistent insomnia that is not resolved by MBTI or CBT-I, then a higher level of mindfulness meditation expertise, BSM expertise (e.g., board certified in behavioral sleep medicine), or sleep medicine expertise (e.g., physician who is board certified in sleep medicine) might be needed. Also, combination approaches using pharmacological and nonpharmacological treatments might be considered throughout this model. Another option is to introduce other delivery methods, such as Internet-based delivery of CBT-I or MBTI. Given that health care is gravitating toward team-based approaches with an emphasis on quality of care and efficiency of health care utilization, this stepped care model might hold promise as a collective method to combat the problem of insomnia as a public health epidemic. This model requires health care providers and policymakers to coordinate their efforts and work together. Perhaps teaching mindfulness principles to these groups can help achieve a mindfulness-based model for health care.

Appendix

The appendix contains materials that can aid instructors in delivering MBTI, including a sample syllabus, handouts, and diaries.

SAMPLE SYLLABUS

Mindfulness-Based Therapy for Insomnia

Welcome to the Mindfulness-Based Therapy for Insomnia (MBTI) program. I am delighted that you have chosen to try something different for treating your insomnia. Over the next 8 weeks, you will be learning different techniques and different ways of thinking about insomnia that we believe will help improve your sleep and your daytime functioning.

Instructor: Jason Ong, PhD

Contact Information: If you have questions or concerns, please contact Jason Ong at 123-456-7890.

Program Requirements: To maximize our ability to help you and to learn from you, we expect you to be committed to this program. We expect you to practice the meditations and sleep recommendations that will be discussed throughout the program. We also expect that you complete the daily diaries on your sleep and meditation. We understand that everyone has a busy schedule, but we believe that a strong commitment and openness to this program will give you the best chance for success.

Program Schedule: The group will meet on Wednesdays from 6:30 p.m. to 9:00 p.m. in Room 123 of the University Medical Center. Please plan to arrive a few minutes early so that you can prepare your mind and body and we can be ready to start on time. The schedule below will provide the dates of each session and the theme of the session:

September 7: Session 1—Introduction and Overview of Program
September 14: Session 2—Stepping Out of "Automatic Pilot"
September 21: Session 3—Paying Attention to Sleepiness and Wakefulness
September 28: Session 4—Working With Sleeplessness at Night
October 5: Session 5—The Territory of Insomnia
October 12: Session 6—Acceptance and Letting Go
October 16: MBTI Retreat
October 19: Session 7—Your Relationship With Sleep
October 26: Session 8—Living Mindfully Beyond MBTI

Absence From Class: If you know in advance that you will not be able to make a class, please contact Dr. Ong to make arrangements to receive the class materials.

HANDOUT 1

Applying Mindfulness Principles to Sleep

In the spirit of cultivating mindfulness, this program will help guide your personal inquiry into your own sleep needs and the optimal state of mind for initiation of sleep (at the beginning or middle of the night). In doing so, you want to bring attention to changing your <u>relationship</u> to sleep rather than to the amount of sleep you get each night. As you begin to change this relationship, you might notice an improvement in the quality of your sleep. Later, you will slowly increase the amount of sleep you get. This approach requires discipline and consistency but follows the principles of mindfulness discussed in this program. These principles can also be applied to sleep:

<u>**Beginner's Mind**</u>: Remember that each night is a new night. Be open and try something different! What you have been doing to this point is probably not working well, so it is time to try something new.

<u>**Nonstriving**</u>: Sleep is a process that cannot be forced but instead should be allowed to unfold. Putting more effort into sleeping longer or better is counterproductive.

<u>**Letting Go**</u>: Attachment to sleep or your ideal sleep needs usually leads to worry about the consequences of sleeplessness. This is counterproductive and inconsistent with the natural process of letting go of the day to allow sleep to come.

<u>**Nonjudging**</u>: It is easy to automatically judge the state of being awake as negative and aversive, especially if you do not sleep well for several nights. However, this negative energy can interfere with the process of sleep. One's relationship to sleep can be a fruitful subject of meditation.

<u>**Acceptance**</u>: Recognizing and accepting your current state is an important first step in choosing how to respond. If you can accept that you are not in a state of sleepiness and sleep is not likely to come soon, why not get out of bed? Many people who have trouble sleeping avoid getting out of bed. Unfortunately, spending long periods of time awake in bed might condition you to being awake instead of asleep in bed.

<u>**Trust**</u>: Trust your sleep system and let it work for you! Trust that your mind and body can self-regulate and self correct for sleep loss. Knowing that short consolidated sleep often feels more satisfying than longer fragmented sleep can help you develop trust in your sleep system. Also, sleep debt can promote good sleep as long as it is not associated with increased effort to sleep.

<u>**Patience**</u>: Be patient! It is unlikely that both the quality and quantity of your sleep will be optimal right away.

These are just some ways that the mindfulness principles are related to sleep. You might discover other connections between these principles and the process of going to sleep or falling back asleep. We encourage you to explore this for yourself and share your experience throughout this program.

HANDOUT 2

Meditation Diary

Please complete the diary for each of your meditation sessions at home. Indicate which type of meditation (sitting, body scan, walking, yoga), the start and end times of your session, and the total minutes spent meditating. Please record each meditation session, even if you practice more than once per day.

Date	Type of meditation (e.g., sitting, body scan, walking)	Session start time	Session end time	Total minutes

HANDOUT 3

Standard Sleep Diary

Consensus Sleep Diary–Core

ID/Name: _____

Today's date	Sample 4/5/11						
1. What time did you get into bed?	10:15 p.m.						
2. What time did you try to go to sleep?	11:30 p.m.						
3. How long did it take you to fall asleep?	55 min.						
4. How many times did you wake up, not counting your final awakening?	3 times						
5. In total, how long did these awakenings last?	1 hour 10 min.						
6. What time was your final awakening?	6:35 a.m.						
7. What time did you get out of bed for the day?	7:20 a.m.						
8. How would you rate the quality of your sleep?	☐ Very poor ☑ Poor ☐ Fair ☐ Good ☐ Very good	☐ Very poor ☐ Poor ☐ Fair ☐ Good ☐ Very good	☐ Very poor ☐ Poor ☐ Fair ☐ Good ☐ Very good	☐ Very poor ☐ Poor ☐ Fair ☐ Good ☐ Very good	☐ Very poor ☐ Poor ☐ Fair ☐ Good ☐ Very good	☐ Very poor ☐ Poor ☐ Fair ☐ Good ☐ Very good	☐ Very poor ☐ Poor ☐ Fair ☐ Good ☐ Very good
9. Comments (if applicable)	I have a cold						

HANDOUT 4

Sleep Hygiene Instructions

The following instructions are intended to improve your sleep hygiene. This is not a quick-fix solution for your insomnia, but following these instructions will minimize habits that are counterproductive for sleep. Please think of this as a first step toward developing awareness of your sleep habits. Later in the program, more specific instructions will be provided that build upon some of these instructions and provide a greater chance to see changes in your sleep patterns.

1. **Be aware of the timing and amount of time spent in bed.** You should regularize the time that you go to bed and get out of bed and also the amount of time you spend in bed.
2. **Be aware of sleep effort.** You should avoid putting effort into trying to sleep. Increased effort to sleep is likely to make you more anxious and frustrated rather than more sleepy.
3. **Monitor intake of substances.** Try to avoid coffee, alcohol, and nicotine starting from the late afternoon or evening. Caffeine is a stimulant that may disrupt normal sleep and can stay in your body for about 4 to 5 hours. It is recommended that you avoid caffeine after about 4 or 5 p.m., depending on your bedtime. Alcoholic beverages can promote relaxation and drowsiness, but the effects of alcohol also disrupt sleep, causing it to become fragmented and restless. For most people, consuming alcohol with dinner is not likely to have a negative impact on sleep, but consuming alcohol 1 to 2 hours prior to bedtime is more likely to have a negative effect on sleep. Nicotine can also have stimulating effects and therefore it is not advisable to use nicotine to help relax at night or to use nicotine when unable to fall back to sleep in the middle of the night.
4. **Regular, moderate exercise can promote sleep over the long run, but attempts to use exercise to "tire oneself to sleep" are not effective.** It is recommended that you continue with your current or planned exercise routine but avoid exercising close to bedtime.
5. **Monitoring eating habits by avoiding late meals.** Digestion is an active process that can cause sleep disruption. It is also not preferable to eat in the middle of the night during prolonged awakenings. However, a light snack at bedtime is not likely to have a negative impact on sleep.
6. **Manage the environment in terms of light, noise, temperature, and safety.** The sleep environment should be comfortable. An eye mask can be used to reduce light exposure. A fan or white noise generator can help to reduce disruptive noise in the environment.

Instructions for the Sleep Consolidation Window

The first recommendation for consolidating your sleep is that you limit the amount of time you stay in bed. This will serve as a "sleep window," or a window of opportunity for sleep to occur. You should begin by allowing yourself a sleep window just slightly more than the amount of actual sleep time that you are currently getting. Although this may sound very drastic, it will quickly help to consolidate your sleep and reduce fragmentation of sleep across a longer time in bed. It can also help you develop a greater awareness of the sensation of sleepiness. Once your sleep is consolidated, you will gradually increase the time you allow yourself to be in bed.

Step 1: Keep a consistent wake-up time. The best way to anchor your biological clock is to adhere to your fixed wake-up time and stick to it every day regardless of how much sleep you actually get on any given night. Get out of bed no later than 15 minutes after your wake-up time. Anchoring your wake-up time is essential for optimal sleep. This practice will help you develop a more stable sleep pattern and will strengthen the natural cues from your internal biological clock that regulates your sleep–wake cycle. An irregular wake-up time can weaken the signal from your biological clock that regulates the timing of your sleep. In fact, you can create the type of sleep problem that occurs in jetlag by varying your wake-up time from day to day. If you stick to a fixed wake-up time you will gradually notice that you become sleepy at roughly the same time most nights, which will eventually allow you to get more sleep and satisfy your sleep need.

Step 2: Establish a window for sleep. Now that you have established a fixed wake-up time, the next step is to figure out how many hours to spend in bed. Looking at your sleep diaries, calculate the average total sleep time (TST) for this last week. Subsequently, your initial time in bed (TIB) is determined using the formula: TIB = average TST + 30 minutes. Adding 30 minutes to the average TST allows for a normal amount of time to fall asleep as well as normal brief awakenings during the night.

Step 3: Determine a recommended bedtime. Using the TIB calculated above, count backwards from your wake-up time. This will be your recommended bedtime. However, it is essential that you consider this recommended bedtime as your **earliest** allowed time to go to bed. It is not required that you go to bed at this time if you do not feel sleepy. Instead, be aware of your state of alertness at this time and **allow yourself to go to bed only if you feel sleepy at this time. If you do not feel sleepy at this time, stay up and wait until you do feel sleepy.** By going to bed only when sleepy you increase the likelihood that you will fall asleep easily. Remember that sleep is an unfolding process. It cannot be forced. Impatience with the natural unfolding of sleep and trying to force sleep to happen are usually not effective or productive. Try practicing nonstriving and letting go of the need to sleep.

Frequently Asked Questions About the Sleep Consolidation Window

My goal is to sleep more! How is setting a shorter sleep window going to help? The first step in the sleep consolidation program is to reduce the amount of time you are lying awake in bed, not to increase the amount of your sleep. As we reduce the wake time in bed, and you gain a better sense of your sleep needs, the window can be widened and you will have an opportunity to get more sleep. Remember, in this program we are trying to let go of the goal to get more sleep!

(continues)

Instructions for the Sleep Consolidation Window

What is the difference between sleepiness and fatigue? Many people misjudge the state of sleepiness. People often confuse the sense of being sleepy with the sense of being fatigued and the desire to rest the mind and the body. The state of being very sleepy is a state of having to struggle to stay awake. When you are close to that state, you are sleepy. In contrast, fatigue usually involves a lack of energy and perhaps some negative reaction, such as frustration or irritability toward this lack of energy. Some people describe this as a "fog," where they are not fully awake but unable to sleep. Becoming aware of the state of your mind and body can help you respond more wisely to sleepiness and fatigue.

Should I have a presleep routine or unwind before my scheduled bedtime? Creating a "buffer zone," or quiet time, for about 30 to 60 minutes prior to your scheduled bedtime can help to prepare your mind for sleep and increase the chances of detecting sleepiness. This time can be spent engaging in activities that are enjoyable on their own, rather than activities that are taken as a means to an end. Usually, soothing activities such as knitting, reading comics, or listening to calming music can be helpful. In contrast, having a rigid routine can sometimes increase anxiety or tension, usually because the routine is used to try and sleep. The practice of nonstriving will help you to shed the day's excitements and tensions, preparing yourself for sleep to unfold.

Can I take a nap during the day? During this period of transition to better sleep, you should generally avoid napping. Sleeping at times other than your sleep window, particularly for more than an hour, might weaken your sleep drive and could undermine the sleep consolidation process. **However, if you find yourself very sleepy** (see above) a brief (20–30 minute) afternoon nap 7 to 9 hours after your morning rise time can be taken to ensure your safety. If you do nap, it is best to nap at approximately the same time daily. Irregular naps may weaken the signal from your biological clock and long naps may weaken your sleep drive. As long as you maintain a consistent wake-up time and follow these recommendations for taking a short nap when needed, it is not likely to interfere with your sleep at night.

Once your sleep consolidation program has been discussed with the instructor, please write down your bedtime and wake time below to help remind you of the plan for the coming week. You might also want to write this on your sleep diary as a reminder.

<u>My Sleep Consolidation Program</u>

For the next week, I should **go to bed no earlier than** _____. However, if I am not sleepy at this time, I should wait until I am aware that the sensation of sleepiness is present.

For the next week, I should **wake up at** _____, regardless of how much sleep I obtained during the night.

HANDOUT 6

Instructions for Adjusting the Sleep Window

The initial sleep window was designed to consolidate your sleep. The best measure of the consolidation of your sleep is sleep efficiency, which is calculated using the following formula:

$$\text{Sleep efficiency} = \frac{\text{Time you actually slept}}{\text{Time you spent in bed}} \times 100$$

A. If your average sleep efficiency is ≥ 90% and you feel that you are not getting a sufficient amount of sleep for optimal functioning during the daytime, increase your sleep window by 15 minutes, at either end of the night. You should stay on the new schedule for at least 7 nights before making changes.
B. If your sleep efficiency is < 80%, decrease your sleep window by 15 minutes, at either end of the night. However, you should not reduce your time in bed below 5 hours. You should stay on the new schedule for at least 7 nights before making changes.
C. If your average sleep efficiency is between 80% and 90% continue on your current sleep window. When your average sleep efficiency does meet Criterion A or Criterion B for 7 consecutive days, you can expand or contract your sleep window according to the instructions above.

Examples:

1. Over the past week, Joe reported an average total sleep time (at night) of 6 hours. Following the sleep consolidation recommendations, he spent an average of 6.5 hours in bed. Therefore, 6 hours (TST)/6.5 hours (TIB) × 100 = 92.3%. With a 92.3% sleep efficiency, Joe is then asked if he has noticed sensations of excessive sleepiness during the day. If so, he can increase his sleep window by 15 minutes to 6.75 hours for the next week.
2. Jane had a rough week and reported an average total sleep time of 5.5 hours over the past week, down from 6.5 hours the previous week. She spent an average of 7 hours in bed hoping to get more sleep. Using the formula, 5.5 / 7 × 100 = 78.6%. With a sleep efficiency of 78.6%, Jane should decrease her sleep window to 6.75 hours for the next week.
3. Over the past week, Jim reported an average total sleep time of 5.75 hours, with some good nights and some bad nights. His sleep window was 7 hours during the past week, for a sleep efficiency of 82.1%. Following the recommendations above, Jim should continue with the same sleep window of 7 hours for the next week.

HANDOUT 7

Sleep Reconditioning Instructions

The instructions below come from behavioral theories of conditioned responses to a certain stimulus. When you go through a period of disturbed sleep, the bed (and bedroom) is no longer associated with the cues that promote sleep. Instead, the bed becomes a place of anxiety, uncertainty, and activation, none of which are conducive to sleep. The basic premise behind these instructions is that if you are in bed and find that you do not feel sleepy, then it is best to get out of sleep mode by sitting up in bed or getting out of bed and moving to another area of the home. Once you are no longer trying to sleep, do a quiet, soothing activity until you regain the sensation of sleepiness. Viewed from the mindfulness perspective, when you become aware that you are not sleepy, instead of striving for a state of sleep, be fully awake. Rather than thinking of this as an unpleasant time, you might think of this as an opportunity to practice mindfulness, something you might not have during the day.

Most importantly, stop trying harder to sleep. This means that it is best to stay out of sleep mode when you are not experiencing the sensation of sleepiness. When you are out of this sleeping position, you should be fully present with whatever activity you do.

Step 1: Become aware of the state of your mind and body. Present-moment awareness is the starting point for choosing how to respond. If you notice that you are tossing and turning and sleep is not happening, pause to recognize your state of mind in the present moment. This might happen at the beginning of the night or if you happen to wake up in the middle of the night. Prolonged periods of being awake in bed usually lead to tossing and turning, becoming frustrated, or worrying about not sleeping, all of which indicates that you are striving for sleep to happen. You might even be excited about something happening in your life. All of these reactions make it difficult to fall asleep. Also, when you lie in bed trying to sleep, wanting and hoping to go back to sleep, you are conditioning yourself to be awake in bed. Recognizing your state of mind and body helps you to determine the next step.

Step 2: Get out of sleep mode. Once you are aware that sleep is not likely to come soon, you can now choose what action to take. **One course of action is to acknowledge this state of wakefulness, get out of bed, and go to another room.** Getting out of bed when you are unable to sleep is not easy. Your bed is comfortable, you might want to get some rest, and you might be hopeful that your continued efforts to sleep will make it happen. However, keep in mind that sleep emerges naturally when the body and the mind are calm and content. Therefore, the activities that you choose to do when you are out of bed should promote that state of mind. Things that are soothing and pleasant usually work well. Many of the same activities that were recommended for the buffer zone (see Handout 5) are also appropriate activities to do here. You might also consider this as an opportunity to practice mindful movement (e.g., walking meditation) or a sitting meditation. Note that if you choose to do this, you should also continue your daytime practice.

If you find that getting out of bed is too difficult or if physical limitations prevent getting out of bed at night, **you can also choose to sit up in bed**. This means getting yourself into an upright position so that your intention is to engage in a soothing activity (as described above) rather than trying to sleep. You might choose to practice a sitting meditation, breathing meditation, or a body scan. Again, you should not use this as a substitute for your daytime practice. Also, if you choose to read, it is better to use a dim light rather than a bright light.

H A N D O U T 7 (*Continued*)

Sleep Reconditioning Instructions

Step 3: Return to a sleeping position only when sleepy. Whatever activity you choose, it is best to **return to a sleeping position when you become aware that you are sleepy**. When you become aware that the mind and body are in a state of calmness, relaxation, and sleepiness, you are more likely to fall asleep. Pay attention to the mind's tendency to want sleep to happen rather than the sensations that naturally arise when sleep is likely to happen.

Frequently Asked Questions

How long should I wait before getting out of bed or sitting up? Generally speaking, when you become aware that sleep is not imminent, you should get out of bed and leave the bedroom. Most people become aware of their nonsleepy state of mind fairly quickly (in less than 15 minutes). Note that we strongly discourage the use of a clock in making this decision because monitoring the clock time could lead to dwelling about not sleeping, which further increases frustration or tension. Instead, be guided by what you have already learned from your mindfulness practice about mental states that are not conducive to sleep. Just learn to calmly observe your state of mind and let it guide you.

How often do I have to follow these instructions? You should follow these instructions every time you become aware of not feeling sleepy while in bed. This should be followed every night and could be more than once per night (e.g., beginning of the night and middle of the night).

Can I still do other activities in bed? While in bed, you should avoid doing things that you do when you are awake. Activities such as watching TV, eating, studying, or talking on the phone should not be done while you are in bed. If you frequently use your bed for activities other than sleep, you are unintentionally training yourself to stay awake in bed. If you avoid these activities while in bed, your bed will eventually become a place where it is easy to go to sleep and stay asleep. Sexual activity is the only exception to this rule. This will help make the bed a strong stimulus (or cue) for sleep. In some situations, such as dorms or studio apartments, you will need to reorganize your room to make a separation between the space you use for sleep and the spaces you use for other activities.

After discussing appropriate soothing activities, please write your choices below.

<u>If I become aware that I am awake and not sleepy in bed, I can choose to</u>

_____

HANDOUT 8

The Nurturing/Depleting Activities Exercise

Instructions: Take a moment to think about the activities that occur on a typical day. What sorts of things do you find yourself doing? Please list all of these activities below.

Morning Activities:

Afternoon Activities:

Evening Activities:

After you have completed your list, go through each activity and write an "N" next to the activities that are "nurturing" and a "D" next to the activities that are "depleting." If an activity can be either N or D, chose what is most typical for you. Finally, tally up how many Ns and Ds you have listed.

Total N Activities: _____   **Total D Activities:** _____

HANDOUT 9

An Action Plan for Working Insomnia

It is important to keep in mind the different aspects of this program that were found to be helpful in working with the entire territory of insomnia. Much like the theme of impermanence discussed throughout this program, sleep disturbance might return in the future. Therefore, it is helpful to have an action plan so that you can be prepared to work with insomnia if it does arrive in the future.

Please answer the questions below by listing what you learned during this program as part of your own action plan for working with the territory of insomnia.

When I notice that my sleep is disturbed, I can bring awareness to

To work with the territory of insomnia, I can choose to respond by

HANDOUT 10

Certificate of Compassion

Certificate of Compassion

is presented to

Insert STUDENT'S NAME here

for

Completion of the Mindfulness-Based Therapy for Insomnia

Signature   Date

References

Adam, K., Tomeny, M., & Oswald, I. (1986). Physiological and psychological differences between good and poor sleepers. *Journal of Psychiatric Research, 20,* 301–316. http://dx.doi.org/10.1016/0022-3956(86)90033-6

American Academy of Sleep Medicine. (2005). *The international classification of sleep disorders* (2nd ed.). Rochester, MN: Author.

American Academy of Sleep Medicine. (2014). *International classification of sleep disorders* (3rd ed.). Darien, IL: Author.

American Psychiatric Association. (2000). *Diagnostic and statistical manual of mental disorders* (4th ed., text rev.). Washington, DC: Author.

American Psychiatric Association. (2013). *Diagnostic and statistical manual of mental disorders* (5th ed.). Arlington, VA: Author.

American Psychological Association. (2010). *Ethical principles of psychologists and code of conduct (2002, Amended June 1, 2010).* Retrieved from http://www.apa.org/ethics/code/index.aspx

Andersen, S. R., Würtzen, H., Steding-Jessen, M., Christensen, J., Andersen, K. K., Flyger, H., . . . Dalton, S. O. (2013). Effect of mindfulness-based stress reduction on sleep quality: Results of a randomized trial among Danish breast cancer patients. *Acta Oncologica, 52,* 336–344. http://dx.doi.org/10.3109/0284186X.2012.745948

Baer, R. A., Smith, G. T., & Allen, K. B. (2004). Assessment of mindfulness by self-report: The Kentucky Inventory of Mindfulness Skills. *Assessment, 11*, 191–206.

Baer, R. A., Smith, G. T., Hopkins, J., Krietemeyer, J., & Toney, L. (2006). Using self-report assessment methods to explore facets of mindfulness. *Assessment, 13*(1), 27–45.

Barks, C. (1995). *The essential Rumi.* New York, NY: HarperCollins.

Barlow, D. H. (2004). *Anxiety and its disorders: The nature and treatment of anxiety and panic.* New York, NY: Guilford Press.

Bastien, C. H., Vallières, A., & Morin, C. M. (2001). Validation of the Insomnia Severity Index as an outcome measure for insomnia research. *Sleep Medicine, 2*, 297–307. http://dx.doi.org/10.1016/S1389-9457(00)00065-4

Beck, A. T., Rush, A. J., Shaw, B. F., & Emery, G. (1979). *Cognitive therapy of depression.* New York, NY: Guilford Press.

Beck, A. T., Steer, R. A., & Carbin, M. G. (1988). Psychometric properties of the Beck Depression Inventory: Twenty-five years of evaluation. *Clinical Psychology Review, 8*, 77–100.

Bertisch, S. M., Wells, R. E., Smith, M. T., & McCarthy, E. P. (2012). Use of relaxation techniques and complementary and alternative medicine by American adults with insomnia symptoms: Results from a national survey. *Journal of Clinical Sleep Medicine, 8*, 681–691.

Black, D. S. (2014). Mindfulness-based interventions: An antidote to suffering in the context of substance use, misuse, and addiction. *Substance Use & Misuse, 49*, 487–491. http://dx.doi.org/10.3109/10826084.2014.860749

Black, D. S., & Fernando, R. (2014). Mindfulness training and classroom behavior among lower income and ethnic minority elementary school children. *Journal of Child and Family Studies, 23*, 1242–1246. http://dx.doi.org/10.1007/s10826-013-9784-4

Black, D. S., O'Reilly, G. A., Olmstead, R., Breen, E. C., & Irwin, M. R. (2015). Mindfulness meditation and improvement in sleep quality and daytime impairment among older adults with sleep disturbances: A randomized clinical trial. *JAMA Internal Medicine, 175*, 494–501. http://dx.doi.org/10.1001/jamainternmed.2014.8081

Bonnet, M. H., & Arand, D. L. (1995). 24-hour metabolic rate in insomniacs and matched normal sleepers. *Sleep, 18*, 581–588.

Bonnet, M. H., & Arand, D. L. (1998). Heart rate variability in insomniacs and matched normal sleepers. *Psychosomatic Medicine, 60*, 610–615. http://dx.doi.org/10.1097/00006842-199809000-00017

Bonnet, M. H., & Arand, D. L. (2010). Hyperarousal and insomnia: State of the science. *Sleep Medicine Reviews, 14*, 9–15. http://dx.doi.org/10.1016/j.smrv.2009.05.002

Bootzin, R. R. (1972, August). *Stimulus control treatment for insomnia.* Paper presented at the 80th Annual Convention of the American Psychological Association, Honolulu, HI.

Bootzin, R. R., Epstein, D., & Wood, J. M. (1991). Stimulus control instructions. In P. J. Hauri (Ed.), *Case studies in insomnia* (pp. 19–28). New York, NY: Plenum Press. http://dx.doi.org/10.1007/978-1-4757-9586-8_2

Bootzin, R. R., & Stevens, S. J. (2005). Adolescents, substance abuse, and the treatment of insomnia and daytime sleepiness. *Clinical Psychology Review, 25,* 629–644. http://dx.doi.org/10.1016/j.cpr.2005.04.007

Borbély, A. A. (1982). A two process model of sleep regulation. *Human Neurobiology, 1,* 195–204.

Borbély, A. A., & Achermann, P. (1999). Sleep homeostasis and models of sleep regulation. *Journal of Biological Rhythms, 14,* 557–568.

Bowen, S., Witkiewitz, K., Dillworth, T. M., Chawla, N., Simpson, T. L., Ostafin, B. D., . . . Marlatt, G. A. (2006). Mindfulness meditation and substance use in an incarcerated population. *Psychology of Addictive Behaviors, 20,* 343–347.

Breslau, N., Roth, T., Rosenthal, L., & Andreski, P. (1996). Sleep disturbance and psychiatric disorders: A longitudinal epidemiological study of young adults. *Biological Psychiatry, 39,* 411–418. http://dx.doi.org/10.1016/0006-3223(95)00188-3

Britton, W. B., Haynes, P. L., Fridel, K. W., & Bootzin, R. R. (2010). Polysomnographic and subjective profiles of sleep continuity before and after mindfulness-based cognitive therapy in partially remitted depression. *Psychosomatic Medicine, 72,* 539–548. http://dx.doi.org/10.1097/PSY.0b013e3181dc1bad

Britton, W. B., Haynes, P. L., Fridel, K. W., & Bootzin, R. R. (2012). Mindfulness-based cognitive therapy improves polysomnographic and subjective sleep profiles in antidepressant users with sleep complaints. *Psychotherapy and Psychosomatics, 81,* 296–304. http://dx.doi.org/10.1159/000332755

Broomfield, N. M., & Espie, C. A. (2005). Towards a valid, reliable measure of sleep effort. *Journal of Sleep Research, 14,* 401–407.

Buck, C. J. (2015). *2016 ICD–10–CM standard edition.* Philadelphia, PA: Elsevier.

Buysse, D. J., Ancoli-Israel, S., Edinger, J. D., Lichstein, K. L., & Morin, C. M. (2006). Recommendations for a standard research assessment of insomnia. *Sleep, 29,* 1155–1173.

Buysse, D. J., Germain, A., Moul, D. E., Franzen, P. L., Brar, L. K., Fletcher, M. E., . . . Monk, T. H. (2011). Efficacy of brief behavioral treatment for chronic insomnia in older adults. *Archives of Internal Medicine, 171,* 887–895. http://dx.doi.org/10.1001/archinternmed.2010.535

Buysse, D. J., Reynolds, C. F., III, Kupfer, D. J., Thorpy, M. J., Bixler, E., Manfredi, R., . . . (1994). Clinical diagnoses in 216 insomnia patients using the International Classification of Sleep Disorders (ICSD), DSM-IV and ICD-10 categories: A report from the APA/NIMH DSM-IV Field Trial. *Sleep, 17,* 630–637.

Buysse, D. J., Reynolds, C. F., III, Monk, T. H., Berman, S. R., & Kupfer, D. J. (1989). The Pittsburgh sleep quality index: A new instrument for psychiatric practice and research. *Psychiatric Research, 28,* 193–213.

Carlson, L. E., Doll, R., Stephen, J., Faris, P., Tamagawa, R., Drysdale, E., & Speca, M. (2013). Randomized controlled trial of mindfulness-based cancer recovery versus supportive expressive group therapy for distressed survivors of breast cancer. *Journal of Clinical Oncology, 31,* 3119–3126. http://dx.doi.org/10.1200/JCO.2012.47.5210

Carlson, L. E., & Garland, S. N. (2005). Impact of mindfulness-based stress reduction (MBSR) on sleep, mood, stress and fatigue symptoms in cancer outpatients. *International Journal of Behavioral Medicine, 12,* 278–285. http://dx.doi.org/10.1207/s15327558ijbm1204_9

Carlson, L. E., & Speca, M. (2010). *Mindfulness-based cancer recovery.* Oakland, CA: New Harbinger.

Carlson, L. E., Speca, M., Patel, K. D., & Goodey, E. (2003). Mindfulness-based stress reduction in relation to quality of life, mood, symptoms of stress, and immune parameters in breast and prostate cancer outpatients. *Psychosomatic Medicine, 65,* 571–581. http://dx.doi.org/10.1097/01.PSY.0000074003.35911.41

Carmody, J. F., Crawford, S., Salmoirago-Blotcher, E., Leung, K., Churchill, L., & Olendzki, N. (2011). Mindfulness training for coping with hot flashes: Results of a randomized trial. *Menopause, 18,* 611–620. http://dx.doi.org/10.1097/gme.0b013e318204a05c

Carney, C. E., Buysse, D. J., Ancoli-Israel, S., Edinger, J. D., Krystal, A. D., Lichstein, K. L., & Morin, C. M. (2012). The consensus sleep diary: Standardizing prospective sleep self-monitoring. *Sleep, 35,* 287–302. http://dx.doi.org/10.5665/sleep.1642

Carney, C. E., & Edinger, J. D. (2006). Identifying critical beliefs about sleep in primary insomnia. *Sleep, 29,* 342–350.

Carskadon, M. A., Dement, W. C., Mitler, M. M., Roth, T., Westbrook, P. R., & Keenan, S. (1986). Guidelines for the Multiple Sleep Latency Test (MSLT): A standard measure of sleepiness. *Sleep, 9,* 519–524.

Collins, B. (2001). *Sailing alone around the room: New and selected poems.* New York, NY: Random House.

Consortium of Academic Health Centers for Integrative Medicine. (2015). *Definition of integrative medicine and health.* Retrieved from https://www.imconsortium.org/about/about-us.cfm

Constantino, M. J., Manber, R., Ong, J., Kuo, T. F., Huang, J. S., & Arnow, B. A. (2007). Patient expectations and therapeutic alliance as predictors of outcome in group cognitive–behavioral therapy for insomnia. *Behavioral Sleep Medicine, 5,* 210–228. http://dx.doi.org/10.1080/15402000701263932

Cullen, M. (2011). Mindfulness-based interventions: An emerging phenomenon. *Mindfulness, 2,* 186–193. http://dx.doi.org/10.1007/s12671-011-0058-1

Daley, M., Morin, C. M., LeBlanc, M., Grégoire, J. P., & Savard, J. (2009). The economic burden of insomnia: Direct and indirect costs for individuals with insomnia syndrome, insomnia symptoms, and good sleepers. *Sleep, 32,* 55–64.

Dalrymple, K. L., Fiorentino, L., Politi, M. C., & Posner, D. (2010). Incorporating principles from acceptance and commitment therapy into cognitive-behavioral therapy for insomnia: A case example. *Journal of Contemporary Psychotherapy, 40,* 209–217. http://dx.doi.org/10.1007/s10879-010-9145-1

Devilly, G. J., & Borkovec, T. D. (2000). Psychometric properties of the credibility/expectancy questionnaire. *Journal of Behavior Therapy and Experimental Psychiatry, 31,* 73–86. http://dx.doi.org/10.1016/S0005-7916(00)00012-4

Edinger, J. D., Means, M. K., Carney, C. E., & Krystal, A. D. (2008). Psychomotor performance deficits and their relation to prior nights' sleep among individuals with primary insomnia. *Sleep, 31,* 599–607.

Edinger, J. D., Wohlgemuth, W. K., Radtke, R. A., Marsh, G. R., & Quillian, R. E. (2001). Cognitive–behavioral therapy for treatment of chronic primary insomnia: A randomized controlled trial. *JAMA, 285,* 1856–1864. http://dx.doi.org/10.1001/jama.285.14.1856

Edinger, J. D., Wyatt, J. K., Stepanski, E. J., Olsen, M. K., Stechuchak, K. M., Carney, C. E., . . . Krystal, A. D. (2011). Testing the reliability and validity of *DSM–IV–TR* and *ICSD–2* insomnia diagnoses. Results of a multitrait-multimethod analysis. *Archives of General Psychiatry, 68,* 992–1002. http://dx.doi.org/10.1001/archgenpsychiatry.2011.64

Epstein, D. R., Sidani, S., Bootzin, R. R., & Belyea, M. J. (2012). Dismantling multicomponent behavioral treatment for insomnia in older adults: A randomized controlled trial. *Sleep, 35,* 797–805. http://dx.doi.org/10.5665/sleep.1878

Espie, C. A. (2002). Insomnia: Conceptual issues in the development, persistence, and treatment of sleep disorder in adults. *Annual Review of Psychology, 53,* 215–243. http://dx.doi.org/10.1146/annurev.psych.53.100901.135243

Espie, C. A., Inglis, S. J., Tessier, S., & Harvey, L. (2001). The clinical effectiveness of cognitive behaviour therapy for chronic insomnia: Implementation and evaluation of a sleep clinic in general medical practice. *Behaviour Research and Therapy, 39,* 45–60. http://dx.doi.org/10.1016/S0005-7967(99)00157-6

Espie, C. A., Kyle, S. D., Williams, C., Ong, J. C., Douglas, N. J., Hames, P., & Brown, J. S. (2012). A randomized, placebo-controlled trial of online cognitive behavioral therapy for chronic insomnia disorder delivered via an automated media-rich web application. *Sleep, 35,* 769–781. http://dx.doi.org/10.5665/sleep.1872

Fernandez-Mendoza, J., Calhoun, S., Bixler, E. O., Pejovic, S., Karataraki, M., Liao, D., . . . Vgontzas, A. N. (2010). Insomnia with objective short sleep duration is associated with deficits in neuropsychological performance: A general population study. *Sleep, 33,* 459–465.

Fichten, C. S., Creti, L., Amsel, R., Bailes, S., & Libman, E. (2005). Time estimation in good and poor sleepers. *Journal of Behavioral Medicine, 28,* 537–553. http://dx.doi.org/10.1007/s10865-005-9021-8

Foley, D., Ancoli-Israel, S., Britz, P., & Walsh, J. (2004). Sleep disturbances and chronic disease in older adults: Results of the 2003 National Sleep Foundation Sleep in America Survey. *Journal of Psychosomatic Research, 56,* 497–502. http://dx.doi.org/10.1016/j.jpsychores.2004.02.010

Ford, D. E., & Kamerow, D. B. (1989). Epidemiologic study of sleep disturbances and psychiatric disorders. An opportunity for prevention? *JAMA, 262,* 1479–1484. http://dx.doi.org/10.1001/jama.1989.03430110069030

Friedman, L., Brooks, J. O., III, Bliwise, D. L., Yesavage, J. A., & Wicks, D. S. (1995). Perceptions of life stress and chronic insomnia in older adults. *Psychology and Aging, 10,* 352–357. http://dx.doi.org/10.1037/0882-7974.10.3.352

Garland, E., Gaylord, S., & Park, J. (2009). The role of mindfulness in positive reappraisal. *EXPLORE: The Journal of Science and Healing, 5,* 37–44. http://dx.doi.org/10.1016/j.explore.2008.10.001

Garland, S. N., Carlson, L. E., Stephens, A. J., Antle, M. C., Samuels, C., & Campbell, T. S. (2014). Mindfulness-based stress reduction compared with cognitive behavioral therapy for the treatment of insomnia comorbid with cancer: A randomized, partially blinded, noninferiority trial. *Journal of Clinical Oncology, 32,* 449–457. http://dx.doi.org/10.1200/JCO.2012.47.7265

Gonzalez-Garcia, M., Ferrer, M. J., Borras, X., Muñoz-Moreno, J. A., Miranda, C., Puig, J., . . . Fumaz, C. R. (2013). Effectiveness of mindfulness-based cognitive therapy on the quality of life, emotional status, and CD4 cell count of patients aging with HIV infection. *AIDS and Behavior, 18,* 676–685. http://dx.doi.org/10.1007/s10461-013-0612-z

Goyal, M., Singh, S., Sibinga, E. M. S., Gould, N. F., Rowland-Seymour, A., Sharma, R., . . . Haythornthwaite, J. A. (2014). Meditation programs for psychological stress and well-being: A systematic review and meta-analysis. *JAMA Internal Medicine, 174,* 357–368. http://dx.doi.org/10.1001/jamainternmed.2013.13018

Gross, C. R., Kreitzer, M. J., Reilly-Spong, M., Wall, M., Winbush, N. Y., Patterson, R., . . . Cramer-Bornemann, M. (2011). Mindfulness-based stress reduction versus pharmacotherapy for chronic primary insomnia: A randomized controlled clinical trial. *EXPLORE: The Journal of Science and Healing, 7,* 76–87. http://dx.doi.org/10.1016/j.explore.2010.12.003

Gross, C. R., Kreitzer, M. J., Russas, V., Treesak, C., Frazier, P. A., & Hertz, M. I. (2004). Mindfulness meditation to reduce symptoms after organ transplant: A pilot study. *Advances in Mind-Body Medicine, 20,* 20–29.

Gross, C. R., Kreitzer, M. J., Thomas, W., Reilly-Spong, M., Cramer-Bornemann, M., Nyman, J. A., . . . Ibrahim, H. N. (2010). Mindfulness-based stress reduction for solid organ transplant recipients: A randomized controlled trial. *Alternative Therapies in Health and Medicine, 16*(5), 30–38.

Hantsoo, L., Khou, C. S., White, C. N., & Ong, J. C. (2013). Gender and cognitive–emotional factors as predictors of pre-sleep arousal and trait hyperarousal in insomnia. *Journal of Psychosomatic Research, 74,* 283–289. http://dx.doi.org/10.1016/j.jpsychores.2013.01.014

Harvey, A. G. (2002). A cognitive model of insomnia. *Behaviour Research and Therapy, 40,* 869–893. http://dx.doi.org/10.1016/S0005-7967(01)00061-4

Hauri, P. (1977). *Current concepts: The sleep disorders.* Kalamazoo, MI: Upjohn.

Hauri, P. (1981). Treating psychophysiologic insomnia with biofeedback. *Archives of General Psychiatry, 38,* 752–758. http://dx.doi.org/10.1001/archpsyc.1981.01780320032002

Hayes, S. C. (2004). Acceptance and commitment therapy and the new behaviour therapies: Mindfulness, acceptance, and relationship. In S. C. Hayes, V. M. Follette, & M. M. Linehan (Eds.), *Mindfulness and acceptance: Expanding the cognitive-behavioral tradition* (pp. 1–29). New York, NY: Guilford Press.

Heidenreich, T., Tuin, I., Pflug, B., Michal, M., & Michalak, J. (2006). Mindfulness-based cognitive therapy for persistent insomnia: A pilot study. *Psychotherapy and Psychosomatics, 75,* 188–189. http://dx.doi.org/10.1159/000091778

Herring, W. J., Snyder, E., Budd, K., Hutzelmann, J., Snavely, D., Liu, K., . . . Michelson, D. (2012). Orexin receptor antagonism for treatment of insomnia: A randomized clinical trial of suvorexant. *Neurology, 79,* 2265–2274. http://dx.doi.org/10.1212/WNL.0b013e31827688ee

Hertenstein, E., Thiel, N., Lüking, M., Külz, A. K., Schramm, E., Baglioni, C., . . . Nissen, C. (2014). Quality of life improvements after acceptance and commitment therapy in nonresponders to cognitive behavioral therapy for primary insomnia. *Psychotherapy and Psychosomatics, 83,* 371–373.

Hofmann, S. G., Sawyer, A. T., & Fang, A. (2010). The empirical status of the "new wave" of cognitive behavioral therapy. *The Psychiatric Clinics of North America, 33,* 701–710. http://dx.doi.org/10.1016/j.psc.2010.04.006

Hofmann, S. G., Sawyer, A. T., Witt, A. A., & Oh, D. (2010). The effect of mindfulness-based therapy on anxiety and depression: A meta-analytic review. *Journal of Consulting and Clinical Psychology, 78,* 169–183. http://dx.doi.org/10.1037/a0018555

Hoge, E. A., Bui, E., Marques, L., Metcalf, C. A., Morris, L. K., Robinaugh, D. J., . . . Simon, N. M. (2013). Randomized controlled trial of mindfulness meditation for generalized anxiety disorder:

Effects on anxiety and stress reactivity. *The Journal of Clinical Psychiatry,* *74,* 786–792. http://dx.doi.org/10.4088/JCP.12m08083

Holbrook, A. M., Crowther, R., Lotter, A., Cheng, C., & King, D. (2000). Meta-analysis of benzodiazepine use in the treatment of insomnia. *Canadian Medical Association Journal, 162,* 225–233.

Hölzel, B. K., Lazar, S. W., Gard, T., Schuman-Olivier, Z., Vago, D. R., & Ott, U. (2011). How does mindfulness meditation work? Proposing mechanisms of action from a conceptual and neural perspective. *Perspectives on Psychological Science, 6,* 537–559. http://dx.doi.org/10.1177/1745691611419671

Huang, W., Kutner, N., & Bliwise, D. L. (2009). A systematic review of the effects of acupuncture in treating insomnia. *Sleep Medicine Reviews, 13,* 73–104. http://dx.doi.org/10.1016/j.smrv.2008.04.002

Hubbling, A., Reilly-Spong, M., Kreitzer, M. J., & Gross, C. R. (2014). How mindfulness changed my sleep: Focus groups with chronic insomnia patients. *BMC Complementary and Alternative Medicine, 14,* 50. http://dx.doi.org/10.1186/1472-6882-14-50

Hughes, J. W., Fresco, D. M., Myerscough, R., van Dulmen, M. H., Carlson, L. E., & Josephson, R. (2013). Randomized controlled trial of mindfulness-based stress reduction for prehypertension. *Psychosomatic Medicine, 75,* 721–728. http://dx.doi.org/10.1097/PSY.0b013e3182a3e4e5

Irwin, M. R. (2015). Why sleep is important for health: A psychoneuroimmunology perspective. *Annual Review of Psychology, 66,* 143–172. http://dx.doi.org/10.1146/annurev-psych-010213-115205

Irwin, M. R., Cole, J. C., & Nicassio, P. M. (2006). Comparative meta-analysis of behavioral interventions for insomnia and their efficacy in middle-aged adults and in older adults 55+ years of age. *Health Psychology, 25,* 3–14.

Irwin, M. R., Olmstead, R., Carrillo, C., Sadeghi, N., Breen, E. C., Witarama, T., . . . Nicassio, P. (2014). Cognitive behavioral therapy vs. Tai Chi for late life insomnia and inflammatory risk: A randomized controlled comparative efficacy trial. *Sleep, 37,* 1543–1552.

Irwin, M. R., Olmstead, R., & Motivala, S. J. (2008). Improving sleep quality in older adults with moderate sleep complaints: A randomized controlled trial of Tai Chi Chih. *Sleep, 3,* 1001–1008.

Jacobs, G. D., Pace-Schott, E. F., Stickgold, R., & Otto, M. W. (2004). Cognitive–behavior therapy and pharmacotherapy for insomnia: A randomized controlled trial and direct comparison. *Archives of Internal Medicine, 164,* 1888–1896. http://dx.doi.org/10.1001/archinte.164.17.1888

Jacobson, E. (1938). *You can sleep well.* New York, NY: McGraw-Hill.

Jansson-Fröjmark, M., & Linton, S. J. (2008). The course of insomnia over one year: A longitudinal study in the general population in Sweden. *Sleep, 31,* 881–886.

Johnson, E. O., Roth, T., & Breslau, N. (2006). The association of insomnia with anxiety disorders and depression: Exploration of the direction of risk. *Journal of Psychiatric Research, 40,* 700–708. http://dx.doi.org/10.1016/j.jpsychires.2006.07.008

Kabat-Zinn, J. (1990). *Full catastrophe living: Using the wisdom of your body and mind to face stress, pain, and illness.* New York, NY: Delacorte Press.

Kabat-Zinn, J., Lipworth, L., Burney, R., & Sellers, W. (1987). Four-year follow-up of a meditation-based program for the self-regulation of chronic pain: Treatment outcomes and compliance. *The Clinical Journal of Pain, 2,* 159–173. http://dx.doi.org/10.1097/00002508-198602030-00004

Kabat-Zinn, J., Wheeler, E., Light, T., Skillings, A., Scharf, M. J., Cropley, T. G., Hosmer, D., & Bernhard, J. D. (1998). Influence of a mindfulness meditation-based stress reduction intervention on rates of skin clearing in patients with moderate to severe psoriasis undergoing photo therapy (UVB) and photochemotherapy (PUVA). *Psychosomatic Medicine, 60,* 625–632. http://dx.doi.org/10.1097/00006842-199809000-00020

Kessler, R. C., Berglund, P. A., Coulouvrat, C., Fitzgerald, T., Hajak, G., Roth, T., . . . Walsh, J. K. (2012). Insomnia, comorbidity, and risk of injury among insured Americans: Results from the America Insomnia Survey. *Sleep, 35,* 825–834. http://dx.doi.org/10.5665/sleep.1884

Khalsa, S. B. S. (2004). Treatment of chronic insomnia with yoga: A preliminary study with sleep–wake diaries. *Applied Psychophysiology and Biofeedback, 29,* 269–278. http://dx.doi.org/10.1007/s10484-004-0387-0

Khoury, B., Lecomte, T., Fortin, G., Masse, M., Therien, P., Bouchard, V., . . . Hofmann, S. G. (2013). Mindfulness-based therapy: A comprehensive meta-analysis. *Clinical Psychology Review, 33,* 763–771. http://dx.doi.org/10.1016/j.cpr.2013.05.005

Klatt, M. D., Buckworth, J., & Malarkey, W. B. (2009). Effects of low-dose mindfulness-based stress reduction (MBSR-ld) on working adults. *Health Education & Behavior, 36,* 601–614. http://dx.doi.org/10.1177/1090198108317627

Koszycki, D., Benger, M., Shlik, J., & Bradwejn, J. (2007). Randomized trial of a meditation-based stress reduction program and cognitive behavior therapy in generalized social anxiety disorder. *Behaviour Research and Therapy, 45,* 2518–2526. http://dx.doi.org/10.1016/j.brat.2007.04.011

Kreitzer, M. J., Gross, C. R., Ye, X., Russas, V., & Treesak, C. (2005). Longitudinal impact of mindfulness meditation on illness burden in solid-organ transplant recipients. *Progress in Transplantation, 15,* 166–172. http://dx.doi.org/10.7182/prtr.15.2.6wx56r4u323851r7

Kristeller, J. L., & Hallett, C. B. (1999). An exploratory study of a meditation-based intervention for binge eating disorder. *Journal of Health Psychology, 4,* 357–363. http://dx.doi.org/10.1177/135910539900400305

Krystal, A. D., Walsh, J. K., Laska, E., Caron, J., Amato, D. A., Wessel, T. C., & Roth, T. (2003). Sustained efficacy of eszopiclone over 6 months of nightly treatment: Results of a randomized, double-blind, placebo-controlled study in adults with chronic insomnia. *Sleep, 26*, 793–799.

Kuisk, L. A., Bertelson, A. D., & Walsh, J. K. (1989). Presleep cognitive hyperarousal and affect as factors in objective and subjective insomnia. *Perceptual and Motor Skills, 69*, 1219–1225. http://dx.doi.org/10.2466/pms.1989.69.3f.1219

Kyle, S. D., Morgan, K., Spiegelhalder, K., & Espie, C. A. (2011). No pain, no gain: An exploratory within-subjects mixed-methods evaluation of the patient experience of sleep restriction therapy (SRT) for insomnia. *Sleep Medicine, 12*, 735–747. http://dx.doi.org/10.1016/j.sleep.2011.03.016

Lazarus, R. S., & Folkman, S. (1984). *Stress, appraisal, and coping.* New York, NY: Springer.

LeBlanc, M., Mérette, C., Savard, J., Ivers, H., Baillargeon, L., & Morin, C. M. (2009). Incidence and risk factors of insomnia in a population-based sample. *Sleep, 32*, 1027–1037.

Lengacher, C. A., Reich, R. R., Post-White, J., Moscoso, M., Shelton, M. M., Barta, M., . . . Budhrani, P. (2012). Mindfulness based stress reduction in post-treatment breast cancer patients: An examination of symptoms and symptom clusters. *Journal of Behavioral Medicine, 35*, 86–94. http://dx.doi.org/10.1007/s10865-011-9346-4

Lichstein, K. L., Durrence, H. H., Taylor, D. J., Bush, A. J., & Riedel, B. W. (2003). Quantitative criteria for insomnia. *Behaviour Research and Therapy, 41*, 427–445. http://dx.doi.org/10.1016/S0005-7967(02)00023-2

Lineberger, M. D., Carney, C. E., Edinger, J. D., & Means, M. K. (2006). Defining insomnia: Quantitative criteria for insomnia severity and frequency. *Sleep, 29*, 479–485.

Lipsky, M. S., & Sharp, L. K. (2001). From idea to market: The drug approval process. *The Journal of the American Board of Family Practice, 14*, 362–367.

Lundh, L. G., & Broman, J. E. (2000). Insomnia as an interaction between sleep-interfering and sleep-interpreting processes. *Journal of Psychosomatic Research, 49*, 299–310. http://dx.doi.org/10.1016/S0022-3999(00)00150-1

Manconi, M., Ferri, R., Sagrada, C., Punjabi, N. M., Tettamanzi, E., Zucconi, M., . . . Ferini-Strambi, L. (2010). Measuring the error in sleep estimation in normal subjects and in patients with insomnia. *Journal of Sleep Research, 19*, 478–486. http://dx.doi.org/10.1111/j.1365-2869.2009.00801.x

Marques, D. R., Gomes, A. A., Clemente, V., dos Santos, J. M., & Castelo-Branco, M. (2015). Default-mode network activity and its role in comprehension and management of psychophysiological insomnia: A new perspective. *New Ideas in Psychology, 36*, 30–37. http://dx.doi.org/10.1016/j.newideapsych.2014.08.001

McCullough, J. P. (2003). *Treatment for chronic depression: Cognitive behavioral analysis system of psychotherapy (CBASP)*. New York, NY: Guilford Press.

Merica, H., Blois, R., & Gaillard, J. M. (1998). Spectral characteristics of sleep EEG in chronic insomnia. *The European Journal of Neuroscience, 10*, 1826–1834. http://dx.doi.org/10.1046/j.1460-9568.1998.00189.x

Morgenthaler, T., Kramer, M., Alessi, C., Friedman, L., Boehlecke, B., Brown, T., . . . American Academy of Sleep Medicine. (2006). Practice parameters for the psychological and behavioral treatment of insomnia: An update. *Sleep, 29*, 1415–1419.

Morin, C. M. (1993). *Insomnia: Psychological assessment and management.* New York, NY: Guilford Press.

Morin, C. M., Bastien, C., & Savard, J. (2003). Current status of cognitive-behavior therapy for insomnia: Evidence for treatment effectiveness and feasibility. In M. L. Perlis & K. L. Lichstein (Eds.), *Treating sleep disorders: Principles and practice of behavioral sleep medicine* (pp. 262–285). Hoboken, NJ: Wiley.

Morin, C. M., Bélanger, L., LeBlanc, M., Ivers, H., Savard, J., Espie, C. A., . . . Grégoire, J. P. (2009). The natural history of insomnia: A population-based 3-year longitudinal study. *Archives of Internal Medicine, 169*, 447–453. http://dx.doi.org/10.1001/archinternmed.2008.610

Morin, C. M., Colecchi, C., Stone, J., Sood, R., & Brink, D. (1999). Behavioral and pharmacological therapies for late-life insomnia: A randomized controlled trial. *JAMA, 281*, 991–999. http://dx.doi.org/10.1001/jama.281.11.991

Morin, C. M., Rodrigue, S., & Ivers, H. (2003). Role of stress, arousal, and coping skills in primary insomnia. *Psychosomatic Medicine, 65*, 259–267. http://dx.doi.org/10.1097/01.PSY.0000030391.09558.A3

Morin, C. M., Stone, J., Trinkle, D., Mercer, J., & Remsberg, S. (1993). Dysfunctional beliefs and attitudes about sleep among older adults with and without insomnia complaints. *Psychology and Aging, 8*, 463–467. http://dx.doi.org/10.1037/0882-7974.8.3.463

National Sleep Foundation. (2002). *Sleep in America poll.* Retrieved from http://sleepfoundation.org/sleep-polls-data/sleep-in-america-poll/2002-adult-sleep-habits

Nicassio, P. M., Mendlowitz, D. R., Fussell, J. J., & Petras, L. (1985). The phenomenology of the pre-sleep state: The development of the pre-sleep arousal scale. *Behaviour Research and Therapy, 23*, 263–271. http://dx.doi.org/10.1016/0005-7967(85)90004-X

Nishino, S., Ripley, B., Overeem, S., Lammers, G. J., & Mignot, E. (2000). Hypocretin (orexin) deficiency in human narcolepsy. *The Lancet, 355*, 39–40. http://dx.doi.org/10.1016/S0140-6736(99)05582-8

Nofzinger, E. A., Buysse, D. J., Germain, A., Price, J. C., Miewald, J. M., & Kupfer, D. J. (2004). Functional neuroimaging evidence for hyperarousal in insomnia. *The American Journal of Psychiatry, 161*, 2126–2128. http://dx.doi.org/10.1176/appi.ajp.161.11.2126

Ohayon, M. M. (2002). Epidemiology of insomnia: What we know and what we still need to learn. *Sleep Medicine Reviews, 6,* 97–111. http://dx.doi.org/10.1053/smrv.2002.0186

Ohayon, M. M., & Roth, T. (2003). Place of chronic insomnia in the course of depressive and anxiety disorders. *Journal of Psychiatric Research, 37,* 9–15. http://dx.doi.org/10.1016/S0022-3956(02)00052-3

Ohayon, M. M., Zulley, J., Guilleminault, C., Smirne, S., & Priest, R. G. (2001). How age and daytime activities are related to insomnia in the general population: Consequences for older people. *Journal of the American Geriatrics Society, 49,* 360–366. http://dx.doi.org/10.1046/j.1532-5415.2001.49077.x

Ong, J., & Sholtes, D. (2010). A mindfulness-based approach to the treatment of insomnia. *Journal of Clinical Psychology, 66,* 1175–1184. http://dx.doi.org/10.1002/jclp.20736

Ong, J. C., Cardé, N. B., Gross, J. J., & Manber, R. (2011). A two-dimensional approach to assessing affective states in good and poor sleepers. *Journal of Sleep Research, 20,* 606–610.

Ong, J. C., Kuo, T. F., & Manber, R. (2008). Who is at risk for drop-out from group cognitive-behavior therapy for insomnia? *Journal of Psychosomatic Research, 64,* 419–425. http://dx.doi.org/10.1016/j.jpsychores.2007.10.009

Ong, J. C., Manber, R., Segal, Z., Xia, Y., Shapiro, S., & Wyatt, J. K. (2014). A randomized controlled trial of mindfulness meditation for chronic insomnia. *Sleep, 37,* 1553–1563. http://dx.doi.org/10.5665/sleep.4010

Ong, J. C., Shapiro, S. L., & Manber, R. (2008). Combining mindfulness meditation with cognitive-behavior therapy for insomnia: A treatment-development study. *Behavior Therapy, 39,* 171–182. http://dx.doi.org/10.1016/j.beth.2007.07.002

Ong, J. C., Shapiro, S. L., & Manber, R. (2009). Mindfulness meditation and cognitive behavioral therapy for insomnia: A naturalistic 12-month follow-up. *EXPLORE: The Journal of Science and Healing, 5,* 30–36. http://dx.doi.org/10.1016/j.explore.2008.10.004

Ong, J. C., Ulmer, C. S., & Manber, R. (2012). Improving sleep with mindfulness and acceptance: A metacognitive model of insomnia. *Behaviour Research and Therapy, 50,* 651–660. http://dx.doi.org/10.1016/j.brat.2012.08.001

Ong, J. C., Wickwire, E., Southam-Gerow, M. A., Schumacher, J. A., & Orsillo, S. (2008). Developing cognitive–behavioral treatments: A primer for early career psychologists. *Behavior Therapist, 31,* 73–77.

Orsillo, S. M., Roemer, L., Lerner, J. B., & Tull, M. T. (2004). Acceptance, mindfulness, and cognitive-behavior therapy: Comparisons, contrasts, and application to anxiety. In S. C. Hayes, V. M. Folette, & M. M. Linehan (Eds.), *Mindfulness and acceptance: Expanding the cognitive-behavioral tradition* (pp. 66–95). New York, NY: Guilford Press.

Parswani, M. J., Sharma, M. P., & Iyengar, S. (2013). Mindfulness-based stress reduction program in coronary heart disease: A randomized control trial. *International Journal of Yoga, 6,* 111–117. http://dx.doi.org/10.4103/0973-6131.113405

Pearson, N. J., Johnson, L. L., & Nahin, R. L. (2006). Insomnia, trouble sleeping, and complementary and alternative medicine: Analysis of the 2002 national health interview survey data. *Archives of Internal Medicine, 166,* 1775–1782. http://dx.doi.org/10.1001/archinte.166.16.1775

Perlis, M. L., Giles, D. E., Mendelson, W. B., Bootzin, R. R., & Wyatt, J. K. (1997). Psychophysiological insomnia: The behavioural model and a neurocognitive perspective. *Journal of Sleep Research, 6,* 179–188. http://dx.doi.org/10.1046/j.1365-2869.1997.00045.x

Riemann, D., Spiegelhalder, K., Feige, B., Voderholzer, U., Berger, M., Perlis, M., & Nissen, C. (2010). The hyperarousal model of insomnia: A review of the concept and its evidence. *Sleep Medicine Reviews, 14,* 19–31. http://dx.doi.org/10.1016/j.smrv.2009.04.002

Rounsaville, B. J., Carroll, K. M., & Onken, L. S. (2001). A stage model of behavioral therapies research: Getting started and moving on from stage I. *Clinical Psychology: Science and Practice, 8,* 133–142. http://dx.doi.org/10.1093/clipsy.8.2.133

Schmidt, S., Grossman, P., Schwarzer, B., Jena, S., Naumann, J., & Walach, H. (2011). Treating fibromyalgia with mindfulness-based stress reduction: Results from a 3-armed randomized controlled trial. *Pain, 152,* 361–369. http://dx.doi.org/10.1016/j.pain.2010.10.043

Schutte-Rodin, S., Broch, L., Buysse, D., Dorsey, C., & Sateia, M. (2008). Clinical guideline for the evaluation and management of chronic insomnia in adults. *Journal of Clinical Sleep Medicine, 4,* 487–504.

Segal, Z. V., Bieling, P., Young, T., MacQueen, G., Cooke, R., Martin, L., . . . Levitan, R. D. (2010). Antidepressant monotherapy vs. sequential pharmacotherapy and mindfulness-based cognitive therapy, or placebo, for relapse prophylaxis in recurrent depression. *Archives of General Psychiatry, 67,* 1256–1264. http://dx.doi.org/10.1001/archgenpsychiatry.2010.168

Segal, Z. V., Williams, J. M. G., & Teasdale, J. D. (2002). *Mindfulness-based cognitive therapy for depression: A new approach to preventing relapse.* New York, NY: Guilford Press.

Shapiro, S. L., Bootzin, R. R., Figueredo, A. J., Lopez, A. M., & Schwartz, G. E. (2003). The efficacy of mindfulness-based stress reduction in the treatment of sleep disturbance in women with breast cancer: An exploratory study. *Journal of Psychosomatic Research, 54,* 85–91. http://dx.doi.org/10.1016/S0022-3999(02)00546-9

Shapiro, S. L., Carlson, L. E., Astin, J. A., & Freedman, B. (2006). Mechanisms of mindfulness. *Journal of Clinical Psychology, 62,* 373–386. http://dx.doi.org/10.1002/jclp.20237

Shekleton, J. A., Flynn-Evans, E. E., Miller, B., Epstein, L. J., Kirsch, D., Brogna, L. A., . . . Rajaratnam, S. M. (2014). Neurobehavioral performance impairment in insomnia: Relationships with self-reported sleep and daytime functioning. *Sleep, 37,* 107–116.

Shen, J., Barbera, J., & Shapiro, C. M. (2006). Distinguishing sleepiness and fatigue: Focus on definition and measurement. *Sleep Medicine Reviews, 10,* 63–76. http://dx.doi.org/10.1016/j.smrv.2005.05.004

Singareddy, R., Bixler, E. O., & Vgontzas, A. N. (2010). Fatigue or daytime sleepiness? *Journal of Clinical Sleep Medicine, 6,* 405.

Sivertsen, B., Omvik, S., Pallesen, S., Bjorvatn, B., Havik, O. E., Kvale, G., . . . Nordhus, I. H. (2006). Cognitive behavioral therapy vs. zopiclone for treatment of chronic primary insomnia in older adults: A randomized controlled trial. *JAMA, 295,* 2851–2858. http://dx.doi.org/10.1001/jama.295.24.2851

Smith, M. T., Perlis, M. L., Park, A., Smith, M. S., Pennington, J., Giles, D. E., & Buysse, D. J. (2002). Comparative meta-analysis of pharmacotherapy and behavior therapy for persistent insomnia. *The American Journal of Psychiatry, 159,* 5–11. http://dx.doi.org/10.1176/appi.ajp.159.1.5

Spielman, A. J., Caruso, L. S., & Glovinsky, P. B. (1987). A behavioral perspective on insomnia treatment. *The Psychiatric Clinics of North America, 10,* 541–553.

Spielman, A. J., Saskin, P., & Thorpy, M. J. (1987). Treatment of chronic insomnia by restriction of time in bed. *Sleep, 10,* 45–56.

Stahl, B., & Goldstein, E. (2010). *A mindfulness-based stress reduction workbook.* Oakland, CA: New Harbinger Publications.

Stepanski, E., Zorick, F., Roehrs, T., Young, D., & Roth, T. (1988). Daytime alertness in patients with chronic insomnia compared with asymptomatic control subjects. *Sleep, 11,* 54–60.

Stepanski, E. J., & Wyatt, J. K. (2003). Use of sleep hygiene in the treatment of insomnia. *Sleep Medicine Reviews, 7,* 215–225. http://dx.doi.org/10.1053/smrv.2001.0246

Tang, N. K., & Harvey, A. G. (2005). Time estimation ability and distorted perception of sleep in insomnia. *Behavioral Sleep Medicine, 3,* 134–150. http://dx.doi.org/10.1207/s15402010bsm0303_2

Taylor, D. J., Mallory, L. J., Lichstein, K. L., Durrence, H. H., Riedel, B. W., & Bush, A. J. (2007). Comorbidity of chronic insomnia with medical problems. *Sleep, 30,* 213–218.

Taylor, D. J., Perlis, M. L., McCrae, C. S., & Smith, M. T. (2010). The future of behavioral sleep medicine: A report on consensus votes at the Ponte Vedra Behavioral Sleep Medicine Consensus Conference, March 27–29, 2009. *Behavioral Sleep Medicine, 8,* 63–73. http://dx.doi.org/10.1080/15402001003622776

Taylor, H. L., Hailes, H. P., & Ong, J. (2015). Third-wave therapies for insomnia. *Current Sleep Medicine Reports, 1,* 166–176. http://dx.doi.org/10.1007/s40675-015-0020-1

Teasdale, J. D. (1999). Metacognition, mindfulness and the modification of mood disorders. *Clinical Psychology & Psychotherapy, 6,* 146–155. http://dx.doi.org/10.1002/(SICI)1099-0879(199905)6:2<146:: AID-CPP195>3.0.CO;2-E

van Son, J., Nyklícek, I., Pop, V. J., Blonk, M. C., Erdtsieck, R. J., Spooren, P. F., . . . Pouwer, F. (2013). The effects of a mindfulness-based intervention on emotional distress, quality of life, and HbA(1c) in outpatients with diabetes (DiaMind): A randomized controlled trial. *Diabetes Care, 36,* 823–830. http://dx.doi.org/10.2337/dc12-1477

Vgontzas, A. N., Liao, D., Bixler, E. O., Chrousos, G. P., & Vela-Bueno, A. (2009). Insomnia with objective short sleep duration is associated with a high risk for hypertension. *Sleep, 32,* 491–497.

Vgontzas, A. N., Tsigos, C., Bixler, E. O., Stratakis, C. A., Zachman, K., Kales, A., . . . Chrousos, G. P. (1998). Chronic insomnia and activity of the stress system: A preliminary study. *Journal of Psychosomatic Research, 45,* 21–31.

Witkiewitz, K., Marlatt, G. A., & Walker, D. (2005). Mindfulness-based relapse prevention for alcohol and substance use disorders. *Journal of Cognitive Psychotherapy, 19,* 211–228. http://dx.doi.org/10.1891/jcop.2005.19.3.211

Wyatt, J. K., Cvengros, J. A., & Ong, J. C. (2012). Clinical assessment of sleep–wake complaints. In C. M. Morin & C. A. Espie (Eds.), *The Oxford handbook of sleep and sleep disorders* (pp. 383–404). New York, NY: Oxford University Press.

Yeung, W. F., Chung, K. F., Zhang, S. P., Yap, T. G., & Law, A. C. (2009). Electroacupuncture for primary insomnia: A randomized controlled trial. *Sleep, 32,* 1039–1047.

Yook, K., Lee, S. H., Ryu, M., Kim, K. H., Choi, T. K., Suh, S. Y., . . . Kim, M. J. (2008). Usefulness of mindfulness-based cognitive therapy for treating insomnia in patients with anxiety disorders: A pilot study. *Journal of Nervous and Mental Disease, 196,* 501–503. http://dx.doi.org/10.1097/NMD.0b013e31817762ac

Zammit, G., Erman, M., Wang-Weigand, S., Sainati, S., Zhang, J., & Roth, T. (2007). Evaluation of the efficacy and safety of Ramelteon in subjects with chronic insomnia. *Journal of Clinical Sleep Medicine, 3,* 495–504.

Zernicke, K. A., Campbell, T. S., Blustein, P. K., Fung, T. S., Johnson, J. A., Bacon, S. L., & Carlson, L. E. (2013). Mindfulness-based stress reduction for the treatment of irritable bowel syndrome symptoms: A randomized wait-list controlled trial. *International Journal of Behavioral Medicine, 20,* 385–396. http://dx.doi.org/10.1007/s12529-012-9241-6

Zhang, B., & Wing, Y. K. (2006). Sex differences in insomnia: A meta-analysis. *Sleep, 29,* 85–93.

Zwart, C. A., & Lisman, S. A. (1979). Analysis of stimulus control treatment of sleep-onset insomnia. *Journal of Consulting and Clinical Psychology, 47,* 113–118. http://dx.doi.org/10.1037/0022-006X.47.1.113

Index

after walking meditation, 101
awareness in, 130
body scan, 48, 90–93, 95, 101, 106, 127
breathing meditation, 81, 127
cultivating awareness in, 117
in homework, 124
in program sessions, 101, 109, 120
working through difficult thoughts, emotions, or sensations in, 126

R
Ramelteon, 31–33
Randomized controlled trials
of MBTI, 5–6, 163–169
of MBTs, 169–176
Rapid eye movement (REM) sleep, 33
Reactive mode, 120, 122
Rebound insomnia, 33
Recruitment, patient, 69–71
Recurrent insomnia disorder, 13
Referrals, 153
Reimbursement, for integrative health interventions, 186–187
Relapse prevention, 139–141
Relapse rate, 16
Relationship with sleep, 133–134. *See also* Revisiting the Relationship With Sleep (Session 7)
Relaxation techniques, 43, 46, 48
Relaxation training, 34, 36
Remission rate, 6, 16
Remsberg, S., 35
REM (rapid eye movement) sleep, 33
Research on MBTI, 157–178
acceptance-based strategies vs. MBTI, 176
effectiveness studies, 174
efficacy studies, 5–6, 163–169
future directions for, 176–178
other mindfulness-based approaches vs. MBTI, 169–176
proof-of-concept testing, 159–163
testing for pharmacological treatments vs., 158
Resistance, patient, 147–148, 152–153
Respiration, suppression of, 33
Response bias, 177
Response over time, 18
Retreat, meditation, 142–144, 153, 185
Revisiting the Relationship With Sleep (Session 7), 130–136
didactic portion of, 133–134
homework for, 136
key activities, 75
meditation practice in, 130–133
nurturing/depleting activities exercise in, 135–136
outline, 131
period of inquiry and discussion in, 133
self-compassion in, 134–135
Riedel, B. W., 13
"Right way," demonstrating, 150–151

Rigidity of beliefs, about insomnia, 64–65
Rise time
consistency of, 109, 110
in sleep consolidation program, 103, 104
and timing of circadian rhythm, 55
Rumi, 129
Running, mindful, 133
Rush, A. J., 35

S
Safety behaviors, 65
Santorelli, S. F., 67
Saskin, P., 34
Sawyer, A. T., 46
SBSM (Society of Behavioral Sleep Medicine), 37, 185
Schmidt, S., 171
SE. *See* Sleep efficiency
Secondary arousal, 59–61, 63, 64
Secondary insomnia, 14
Second-order distress, 61, 62
Segal, Z. V., 5, 45–46, 67, 131, 135
Self-compassion
in loving-kindness meditation, 144–146
in mindfulness, 42, 57
in mindfulness meditation, 43–45
in Session 7, 134–135
Self-guided meditation, 120, 121
Self-hatred, 146
Self-monitoring control, 5–6, 163–169
Self-reported measures, of sleepiness and fatigue, 23
Sensation(s)
of sleepiness, 101–102, 114, 115, 122
working through difficult, 126
Sensitive information, sharing of, 149
Shapiro, S. L., 5, 58–59, 159–163, 170
Sharing, in closing ceremony, 141–142
Shaw, B. F., 35
Shifting, metacognitive. *See* Metacognitive shifting
Sholtes, D., 128–129
Short sleep duration, 18
Side effects
of behavioral treatments, 36
of CBT-I, 36–37
of prescription sleep medications, 31, 32
of sleep restriction therapy, 103
Silence, noble, 142, 143
Sitting meditation, 44
as homework, 87, 116
introducing patients to, 81, 82
in opening practice, 88–89, 120, 138
preference for walking meditation vs., 101
Skepticism, about MBTI, 76, 77
Sleep. *See also* Attachment to sleep; Revisiting the Relationship With Sleep (Session 7)
applying mindfulness principles to, 191
during body scan meditation, 91
as essential part of life, 3

About the Author

Jason C. Ong, PhD, is an associate professor in the department of neurology at Northwestern University Feinberg School of Medicine. He is the director of the behavioral sleep medicine training program and the principal investigator of the behavioral sleep and circadian medicine laboratory. He received his doctorate in psychology from Virginia Commonwealth University and completed a fellowship in behavioral sleep medicine at Stanford University School of Medicine. His primary research and clinical interests are behavioral and mindfulness-based treatments for insomnia and other sleep disorders. Other research interests include the impact of sleep disturbance on chronic health conditions.